Research Impact

Hugh P. McKenna

Research Impact

Guidance on Advancement, Achievement and Assessment

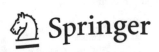 Springer

Hugh P. McKenna (iD)
Ulster University
Ulster
UK

ISBN 978-3-030-57027-9   ISBN 978-3-030-57028-6   (eBook)
https://doi.org/10.1007/978-3-030-57028-6

This Springer imprint is published by the registered company Springer Nature Switzerland AG
The registered company address is: Gewerbestrasse 11, 6330 Cham, Switzerland

Preface

No researcher wants to see the results of their investigations languishing on library shelves or being unknown by their peers and those who would benefit from the findings. Rather, they want to see their research having impact on society, the economy, culture, health or quality of life. Furthermore, high-quality research cannot be done without funding, and more and more funding bodies are focusing their grants on research that is potentially impactful. In addition, for almost 30 years, publicly funded research in the UK has been assessed for quality in a series of research assessment exercises. The most recent one is called the Research Excellence Framework (HEFCE, 2014). As a result of the many reviews of research impact generally and the REF 2014 specifically, this information is in the public domain, and suitable references will be included as signposts for those readers who seek more in-depth information.

Such exercises are also carried out in many countries across the world. These include Finland, Norway, Sweden, Denmark, Holland, Italy, New Zealand, Australia, Romania, Hong Kong, Germany and most recently the Czech Republic. The results are mainly used to inform the allocation of public funding for research and provide accountability for tax payers' money. Increasingly, these exercises are including the assessment of research impact because governments believe it is not unreasonable to ask those whose research work is undertaken at public expense to account for and provide some evidence of their impact.

However, the traditional approach to assuring and assessing the quality of university research has been through quantitative measures such as publications, citations, Ph.D. completions and research income. These are deeply incorporated in the recruitment, retention and reward system for academic staff. It is a truism that research that is published in the top journals and highly cited has benefits for individual researchers but is less beneficial for society. As research impact becomes more important globally, the traditional metrics are beginning to be regarded as only providing a partial picture of full academic impact.

Furthermore, the lessons learned over the last decade in the UK are applicable and transferable to other countries. These are dealt with in this textbook and include how to engage with external stakeholders to ensure the creation of impact, how universities prepare for the assessment of their research impact and how expert panel assessors actually review research impact. The core of research impact assessment is the case study, and a substantial part of Chap. 8 is devoted on how these should be written.

The generation of research impact is complex and resource intensive. This textbook explores these challenges in detail and where possible proposes solutions. There is also a strong link between evidence-informed policy and practice and research impact. This link is analysed and clarification provided on the way forward. Perhaps one of the most difficult ways to create research impact is through public engagement and networking with policy makers. These are highlighted and suggestions for improvement proffered. An overview of how research impact is evaluated in other countries is also presented with lessons that can be disseminated globally.

The research impact agenda is with us and is not going to go away. In fact, it will play a greater role in further research assessment exercises and in research grant applications. It encourages researchers to think more about maximising the benefits of their research, and no reasonable person would deny that this is a good thing. This is the reason why it has been embraced by most academics, universities and governments. I predict that in the years to come more countries will be including research impact assessment in their review of research quality.

I would like to acknowledge the Research Impact Manager and Research Impact Officers at Ulster University. Furthermore, I am grateful to all those workshop delegates whose perceptive questions over the years have had the desired ripple effect in developing my thinking about research impact. My gratitude also goes to Karthik Periyasamy and Nathalie L'Horset-Poulain from Springer who have been unstinting in their positive support and thoughtful advice. Finally, my thanks to members of the REF team at HEFCE and Research England who stimulated my interest in this topic over the past decade.

In all the various international research evaluation exercises, different disciplines and expert panel may have subtle variations in how assessment is undertaken. This textbook takes a general approach; it is highly recommended that those who want more granular details refer to the official guidance. Finally, I want to state that apart from the sources referenced, all the opinions, views and assertions are mine alone. This also includes any errors in content and stylistic inaccuracies. I am not representing Research England or any other government body regionally, nationally or internationally. The next REF has been severely affected by the Covid-19 pandemic. This has affected key deadline dates regarding the submission and assessment of research impact; these new dates have been included in Chap. 2.

Ulster, UK   Hugh P. McKenna

Contents

About the Author

Hugh P. McKenna is a general and psychiatric nurse by background and is currently Dean of Medical School Development at Ulster University. Prior to this, he was in PVC Research and Innovation at Ulster University. He has over 250 publications, including 16 books. He was awarded Commander of the British Empire (CBE) for his work on health and community and is a Fellow of four prestigious organisations. In 2013, he was presented with the Outstanding Achievement Award by the Royal College of Nursing, and in 2014, he received a lifetime achievement Award at the Institute of Psychiatry. In a 2018 UK Government report, he was named as one of the 70 most influential nurses in the 70-year history of the NHS.

Currently, he is an Adjunct/Visiting Professor in universities in Slovenia and Australia. He chairs the same panel for REF 2021. He has also chaired a clinical health research quality panel for the Swedish Research Council and panels for the Hong Kong Council for Accreditation. He is chair of Inspire Wellbeing, the largest mental health, learning disability and addiction charity on the island of Ireland. Recently he received Honorary Doctorates from Edinburgh Napier University and the University of Maribor.

In 2019, he was appointed as a Member of the Academia Europaea, founded as an initiative of The Royal Society to be the official scientific advisory body for the EU. He is a non-executive director on a large health and social care trust in Northern Ireland and is a Trustee for Alzheimer's Society, UK. Until recently, he chaired the Research Committee of the Patient and Client Council.

He chairs the 2021 UK's Research Excellence Framework's (REF) panel for nursing, allied health professions, pharmacy and dentistry. Previously, he chaired the same panel for REF 2014 and one in the 2008 UK Research Assessment Exercise (RAE). He has chaired an equivalent panel for the Swedish Research Council and has inputted into similar exercises in Hong Kong and Australia. He has a unique insight into what research impact is, how it is achieved and assessed and how and where it can have the most benefit.

Research Impact: The What, Why, When and How

1

We grow no food on campus, so like every poet, priest or potter..., we must explain why we have faith in the usefulness of what we do provide (Gray and Gray [1]).

1.1 Introduction

The Cambridge English Dictionary [2] defined impact as '*a powerful effect that something, especially something new, has on a situation or person*'. Alternatively, The Collin's Business Dictionary [3] defined it as *a measure of the tangible and intangible effects (consequences) of one's action or influence upon another*. Therefore, impact is the result of an action or an influence on people or things.

Moving onto research impact, it refers to any type of output of research activities which can be considered to have a 'positive return' for the scientific community, health systems, patients and the society in general [4]. They maintain that it can be grouped into five categories: 'advancing knowledge', 'capacity building', 'informing decision-making', 'health benefits' and 'bro*ad socio-economic benefits*'.

Yet another definition stated that "research impact is the demonstrable contribution that excellent research makes to society and the economy through creating and sharing new knowledge and innovation; inventing ground-breaking new products, companies and jobs; developing new and improving existing public services and policy; enhancing quality of life and health; and many more" [5]. From these definitions, we can extrapolate that research impact is the benefit, effect or change on a variety of people and things, including the economy, society, culture, health or quality of life, as a result of the influence or action of implementing research findings.

But have researchers always seen the pursuit of research impact as their role? Most tend to be very good at investigating the phenomena that are of interest in their field and in answering interesting research questions. They are also adept at disseminating their findings in the form of academic outputs such as papers, books and reports. Most are also active in presenting their research results at international meetings, conferences and exhibitions. Readers will agree that these are laudable endeavours and may create 'academic impact'. However, what researchers are less good at is ensuring that there is uptake and implementation of their research results so as to demonstrate what may be termed 'societal impact'.

H. P. McKenna, *Research Impact*, https://doi.org/10.1007/978-3-030-57028-6_1

1.1.1 Reactive Approach to Research Impact

In this textbook, research impact is synonymous with a benefit or change. This includes producing a benefit by stopping or starting some action or intervention. Traditionally, researchers tended to pursue a well-trodden circular Research Activity Pathway where they Obtain a Research Grant → Carry out an Investigation → Produce Papers and Reports → Speak at Conferences → Increase Their Profile in Their Field → Obtain a Further Research Grant; and the circular pathway continues. It is a bonus if some clinician, entrepreneur or manager comes across their research outputs and adopts and applies the findings and as a result creates benefits. This traditional relationship between researchers and impact can best be described as *reactive*.

1.1.2 Active Approach to Research Impact

In more recent years, some researchers have become converts to evidence-informed practice (see Chap. 7) or knowledge and technology transfer activities supported by universities and government funding agencies. This has encouraged academics to take a more *active* approach to the pursuit of research impact. They still follow the Research Activity Pathway, alluded to above. However, after dissemination, they approach external stakeholders such as clinicians, entrepreneurs or managers and seek to persuade them that their research findings may have some beneficial impact.

In this way, they are actively enabling others to realise the impact from the research. In order to have this relationship with, and influence on, external stakeholders, the researchers must 'get out, get known and get in'. But involving external stakeholders after dissemination is often too late in the Research Activity Pathway. If a researcher wishes to alienate a potential external beneficiary, then approaching them at the end of the project to tell them what they need will certainly do that. It is synonymous with seeking the input of a statistician after data are collected, this approach is not likely to be appreciated. Therefore, while this

more active approach is better than the traditional passive approach, it does not go far enough.

1.1.3 Proactive Approach to Research Impact

Increasingly, there is a recognition that researchers need to engage with stakeholders further upstream. Building networks with those who can shape, advise or use your research from early in the process is important. To be serious about achieving impact, more enlightened researchers are taking a *proactive* approach and involving relevant external stakeholders from the start. It is commonplace in modern health research to have statisticians or health economists as core members of research teams. External stakeholders should also be core team members; their role is to identify the best possible pathways to impact and advise the researchers accordingly.

Here the Research Activity Pathway could be more accurately described as: Obtain a Research Grant → Conduct the Research → Disseminate the Findings → Uptake → Implementation → Impact. What makes this a realistic continuum is the involvement of research end-users as partners in every phase.

Therefore, societal impact is a team sport rather than the result of isolated scientific research alone. It is an iterative process of interaction between researchers and external stakeholders, such as technical experts, professional organisations, industry, government and the public at large. At their best, researchers work closely, and indeed co-produce research, with such partner organisations. They often spend months and years getting to know people within business organisations, groups, communities and government bodies. This is research 'by' and 'with' external stakeholders, rather than research 'about', 'to' or 'for' them. This approach ensures that the studies being conducted are relevant to the stakeholders' needs and that the right questions are asked and the right impactful processes are followed.

It is helpful to consider who the relevant individuals, groups and institutions are and take account of their respective interests. The next step is to engage with them to find out what potential benefits or barriers they see with the project. Maintaining continuous engagement with these stakeholders throughout the research journey is advantageous. Encouraging their input at all stages and enabling them to help shape the project will make them more likely to commit to assisting with generating impact.

This proactive approach to research impact provides an important incentive for researchers in all fields to think about how they should engage with those outside of academia who can translate their research into real-world impacts. It does however require upfront investment from researchers and buy-in from external stakeholders. As a result, it is not problem-free. Including an engagement component acknowledges that researchers are not in direct control of whether there will be uptake and implementation of their research findings. There are also conflict of interest questions concerning whether researchers can work with external organisations while evaluating the work of those organisations.

If we take an example of achieving economic impact from research, then the following linear framework shows the essential nature of the partnership between researchers and external stakeholders. The stages are as follows: Research → Disseminating → Design and Engineering → Manufacturing → Marketing → Sales → Benefits for Customers. Within this framework, the active participation of an external partner is crucial to successfully bring the innovation to market. Without this, the research, no matter how good, will have very little impact.

Sometimes, the innovators are the researchers themselves, who establish a university spin-out company. However, in my experience, these start-ups have difficulty in growing without the help of external company directors and venture capitalists. Therefore, in terms of economic impact, the underpinning research may be of the highest quality, but no benefit will accrue without the proactive internal–external partnership. The same principle applies to other types of impact, whether societal, cultural, quality of life or health.

Reflection Point 1.1 Questions Researchers Need to Ask to Create Research Impact
The pro-active approach to research impact has encouraged researchers to ask themselves perceptive questions. Readers are asked to consider what those questions might be. Perhaps some of the following are pertinent:

- Who are the actual and potential research users?
- Who, among your colleagues, are already working with them?
- Where are the actual and potential research users?
- When in the best time to engage with them?
- What are their interests, priorities and needs?
- What is in it for them; how will they benefit?
- What are your objectives from this engagement?
- What methods will you use to access and engage with them?
- What resources will you need to create meaningful engagement?
- How do you align your objectives with their priorities?
- What are the main barriers to successful engagement?
- How do you ensure long-term engagement?

See Appendix A.

Therefore, to take a proactive approach to research impact not only requires a change of researcher mind set, it also requires a change of culture. The following section discusses the reasons for this cultural change.

1.2   Why Is Research Impact Important?

For almost half a century, governments invested public funds in projects with the expectation that military, economic, medical and other benefits would occur. This trend has continued with increasing levels of public money being invested in research. The payback for such expenditure is research impact, and this will be explored below. It is also certain that achieving research impact can be inspiring and informative as well as a cause for celebration. This means it can be exciting for researchers generally and for early career researchers specifically. The following section will seek to provide some answers to why research impact has become so important in the past decade.

1.2.1   Moral Imperative

It is always good to quote Florence Nightingale when reflecting on what health care is for. In 1860 she wrote, 'We must show people how their money is being spent and what amount of good is really being done with it' ([6], p 27). On a similar theme, and 250 years before Nightingale, Francis Bacon (1561–1626) emphasised that the sole purpose of research was to be 'of benefit to man-

kind' [7]. Therefore, when researchers complete their investigations, often at public expense, they need to remember that they have a moral duty not just to share the results with the academic community; they also need to consider how their findings can benefit society. It could be argued that not to do so is unethical. Research subjects and respondents give up valuable time and, in many cases, personal data and insights, to enable researchers to seek answers to their research questions and address their aims and objectives. Because of this, researchers have a responsibility to ensure that the greatest benefits accrue from that voluntary participation.

Furthermore, why do researchers exist and why do governments and other research funding bodies invest considerable resources in scientific investigations? It is to make something better; without this, research is an empty exercise and research for its own sake could also be accused of being immoral. No reasonable person would deny that the global sustainability goals outlined in Fig. 1.1 are critical for the survival of humankind. Who for instance would argue that eradicating poverty is a bad thing or that good health and well-being was not desired or that zero hunger is not a worthwhile pursuit? The role of researchers across the globe is to focus their efforts and have a positive impact on these and other important global problems. To do otherwise, raises impor-

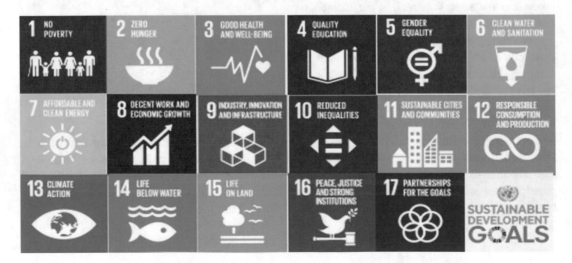

Fig. 1.1   The UN Sustainability Development Goals 2030, as drivers for research impact. [8]

tant moral questions that undermine the goals of research and researchers.

A related reason for creating research impact is personal fulfilment. It is common for researchers to be motivated to generate impact by altruism. They have an inherent desire to ensure that their work adds to the public good; otherwise, why do it at all? This Good Samaritan approach to research impact reflects human nature and the desire to help others. The rewards are many and include increased self-esteem, increased pleasure and increased personal and job satisfaction.

1.2.2   The Role of Universities as Drivers for Impact

In the second half of the nineteenth century, Justus von Liebig, a chemist at the University of Gießen in Germany, established his subject as an academic discipline and gave it a foundation in experimental basic research [9]. He also revolutionised teaching by basing it on laboratory work. The chemists he trained went on to underpin the rise of the dye industry, particularly in Germany. Two of the dye factories that opened in this period remain the beating heart of Germany's chemical and pharmaceutical industry, Bayer and BASF, founded in 1863 and 1865 respectively. They are now global players, each with more than 100,000 employees worldwide and tens of billions in revenues. I provide this example (from many that I could have selected) to illustrate that successful companies often emerge out of collaborations between the industrial and university sectors.

Traditionally, there have been two main funding streams for UK universities. These are the government's annual block grants for teaching and research. Naturally, university leaders have done everything possible to increase their income from these sources. The *Magna Charta Universitatum* was drafted in Bologna in 1988 and signed by all the EU university rectors. It stressed that the two pillars of teaching and research in universities must be inseparable if tuition is not to lag behind changing needs, the demands of society and advances in scientific

knowledge [10]. However, a third stream of university funding appeared, which focused upon knowledge and technology transfer. Subsequently, academic staff, especially from science, engineering and computing departments became involved in intellectual property, patents, licencing and early start companies. Even though the emphasis was on economic generation and growth, it became the forerunner of research impact.

Being near high quality research enables companies to recruit great people and innovate through collaboration, an increasingly common model in everything from biotechnology to computing. A country's science base is an ecosystem of excellent researchers based in academia, in spin-outs, in small- and medium-sized businesses and large research-intensive companies. Such innovation depends on this interconnected system of bright people working together.

Research impact has become an integral part of research life and of universities' reputations and finances. As a sector, it has become accustomed to expectations around generating and showcasing the societal benefit of its research. Such knowledge is accepted as the driver of productivity and economic growth. The term 'knowledge-based economy' stems from this fuller recognition of the place of knowledge and technology in modern economies. Traditionally, universities were perceived as temples of knowledge, often caricatured as ivory towers behind high walls. But in times of economic and social upheaval, governments demand that they become a channel linking the world of knowledge with the world of business. This is not new; in ancient Athens, the Agora, or business unit, was located beside the academy on the slopes of the Acropolis. This was to ensure that there was every opportunity for merchants to meet with scholars and share problems and solutions. Today, this is more important than ever for both society and the universities to thrive.

Universities are seen, and see themselves, as embedded parts of society, hubs around which impact can thrive, connecting smart people and smart ideas, critical to the continuing success of a country's strongest sectors, and constantly pushing at the knowledge frontier. This is not to distort from the university's mission to educate, but to extend it and increase the flow of good ideas into society and the economy, as much as the flow of good people. With their knowledge generation and leadership, universities write themselves into the story of a country's social and economic impact.

Sir Ron Dearing, the author of the Dearing Report into Higher Education ([11]. p 23), stated that 'In the middle ages, the centre of the community was the medieval castle. In the 18th century, it was the mines and manufacturing industries. Today, it is the university'. In fact, the word university derives from the Latin root meaning 'community'. I would argue that not only are our universities at the centre of the community, increasingly they are at the very heart of innovation and impact.

Because of their scale, local rootedness and community links, universities are acknowledged to play a key role in local development and social cohesion and economic growth. They represent the 'sticky capital' that attracts foreign and direct investment and around which economic growth strategies are planned and delivered. The OECD [12] concluded that the primary determinant of growth for developed economies is their level of research and development (R&D) spending. It is public R&D spending that levers in private investment, and the primary focus of public R&D spending is the university. Private companies locate themselves only where there is both existing competitive publicly funded research and development infrastructure and abundant higher-level skills.

In most countries, universities rely on public funding for their teaching and research activities. The *quid pro quo* is that they have to prove their value to society. This is the philosophical basis for the assessment of research impact. It is also indicative of the trend in recent years for university managers and politicians to emphasise the importance of higher education for economic and social regeneration specifically or for wealth creation generally. A commonly held view is that universities should encourage the seamless transfer of knowledge from the research laboratory to the lecture hall to the marketplace, because it is recognised that research drives innovation and innovation feeds productivity, which fuels the creation of wealth and economic growth [13].

The obvious question to end this section is whether research impact is now synonymous with excellence in universities. An article by Baker [14] in the June issues of the *Times Higher Education* analysed the pursuit of excellence in universities. Numerous indicators of excellence were identified, including the usual suspects of citation rankings, international staff and research income. The concept of research impact was not mentioned. He did state that a factor in research excellence is 'industry, social and governmental take-up of research'. However, he refers to Simon Marginson, professor of higher education at the University of Oxford, who maintained that this 'is not so directly driven by an excellence programme, and depends on other conditions' (p. 2). This is disappointing and gives the wrong message to those academics who want their partnership for impact to be recognised as central to university research excellence.

Reflection Point 1.2 Why Should Universities Produce Research Impact?

The Haldane principle is the belief that decisions about what to spend research funds on should be made by researchers rather than government [15]. This posits that universities are independent institutions. Why then should they be mandated by government to generate research impact?

This question is addressed by Penfield et al. [16] who maintained that the reasoning behind the move towards assessing university research impact, while complex, can be justified in four ways:

- It enables universities to monitor and manage their performance and understand and disseminate the contribution that they are making to local, national and international communities.

- It demonstrates to government, stake-holders and the wider public the value of university research funded out of the public purse.
- By assessing the contribution that university research makes to society and the economy, future funding can be allocated where it is perceived to bring about the desired impact.
- It provides understanding on the method and routes by which university research leads to impacts and better ways of delivering impact (p. 24).

Accepting this, university research needs to capture and celebrate its impacts more than ever before. They need to continue to show that science and research make a positive difference to society, culture and the economy. They need to accept that research impact is not a luxury but a necessity for continued government support. The value of university research must continually be 'sold' to governments, and impact is the way for this to be accomplished.

1.2.3   Research Impact as a Dictate from Funding Bodies

Until relatively recently, academic research was judged by an assessment of published peer-reviewed papers. In fact, it has often been said that research is not finished until it is communicated. However, this view is becoming outdated; it is more appropriate now to state that research is not finished until it has changed something for the better; in other words, it needs to have impact. It seems obvious that if funding bodies support high-quality research that addresses important problems, then they would expect that impact would follow.

It is a given that planning for impact is best done at the beginning of the research process. If researchers focus on the impact of their study from the outset, they are more likely to achieve it. To start a project without thinking and planning

for the benefits it will accrue will at best lead to accidental impact or no impact. A question I often ask my PhD students at the start of their course is 'Who or what will benefit from your research study?' If they cannot answer that question, I wonder why they should spend years undertaking their project.

In the last decade, funding bodies began to mandate that researchers identify 'pathways to impact' in their grant proposals. These included the UK Funding Councils (RCUK), the European Union (EU) and charity funders. It was common to see specific impact requirements built into funding calls, making impact an integral part of the application. This was linked to the fact that most research monies come from the public purse in the form of taxes or charitable giving. Also, funding bodies have been enthused by what their research monies can achieve for researchers, for science and for society. It is not surprising that this view from grant awarding bodies incentivised most researchers to take research impact more seriously than they had hitherto.

In March 2020, the United Kingdom Research and Innovation (UKRI), the government research policy and funding body, appeared to reverse the ruling that researchers had to outline pathways to impact in their research bids. The announcement seemed to contradict the UKRI's mission to ensure everyone in society benefits from world-leading research and innovation. Furthermore, this was perceived by some in the research community as a sign of backtracking on the impact agenda and for encouraging researchers to retreat to what they knew best, doing research and disseminating the results. It had the potential to be an own goal by a government committed to deliver an ambitious industrial strategy. But, perhaps driving an impact agenda around pathways to impact on individual projects is not a good strategy. A broader approach focusing on academic-societal engagement and networking might possibly be more successful.

However, shortly after the announcement to end pathways to impact, the UKRI emphasised that the impact agenda remained vital. Researchers will still be encouraged to detail any activities relating to the potential translation of their findings within grant proposals. David Carr, programme manager at The Wellcome Trust, a prestigious UK research funding body, asserted that it was still fundamental to be able to assess inputs and outputs of research and to see its impacts [17]. So instead of there being a tokenistic 'Pathway to Impact' section, some research funders dictate that impact should be embedded throughout the grant proposal. Grant reviewers will be tasked with considering the appropriateness of all the impact activities outlined in the funding bids.

Therefore, the UK government and other grant awarding bodies continue to seek a demonstration of some kind of return on investment. Undoubtedly, impact provides evidence that academic research should continue to be financed and is directly benefitting the taxpayers who fund it. The generation of impact will help the general public better understand the value of the research that they support through their taxes and that charitable donors fund through their giving.

1.2.4 The Research Excellence Framework

When it comes to research, the UK universities are funded on a competitive reward basis; in other words, the best gets the money. Therefore, the greatest driver for research impact has been the way that governments distribute public funding for university research. For example, since 1986, the quality of the structures, processes and outcomes of UK university research have been evaluated in a series of Government Research Assessment Exercises (RAE). Since 2014, these have been designated the Research Excellence Framework (REF). Such assessment exercises are carried out in many countries across the world. This includes France, Finland, Norway, Sweden, Denmark, Holland, Italy, New Zealand, Australia, Romania, Hong Kong, Germany and most recently the Czech Republic. The UK Department for Business, Energy and Industrial Strategy [18] confirmed that many national research assessment systems assess non-academic outputs and socio-economic outcomes

and impacts. Examples of how different countries do this will be described in Chap. 9.

Every 5–6 years, universities in these countries submit elements of their research to expert panels to be assessed for quality. Such submissions are mainly composed of publications and other outputs of research activity. In addition, some include information pertaining to the research environment such as the research strategy, infrastructure, funding, PhD completions, staffing strategy, research esteem and research collaborations.

In the UK, the results of the REF inform the distribution of approximately £2 billion of taxpayers' money to the UK universities in the form of an annual research block grant. It is referred to as Quality Research (QR) funding. Considering that the REF takes place every 5–6 years, the total sum apportioned over that time period is closer to £10–12 billion. This is allocated with very little restrictions on how this money can be spent by university leaders. They are free to deploy it to wherever they believe it will be most effective. It has been used for new departments and institutes, to strategically fund PhD students, for research fellowship schemes, and to pump prime research collaborations with the health service and with business.

QR funding also supports research activities that is not fully funded by other grants. For example, charities fund university research, but they do not pay overheads. When a researcher wins a grant from a charity, QR funding covers the indirect costs of the project such as the salaries of some of the staff working on the project and even the light and heat required for the building. Similarly, when a UK researcher obtains a prestigious Research Council grant, only 75% of the full costs is paid; QR funding covers the 25% shortfall. It is a little-known fact that many of the salaries for full-time researchers in the UK universities are funded out of the QR allocation.

University research is also funded from other sources. For example, industry and business fund university research; however, they tend to support the 'innovation' end of the research continuum because it is closer to market and brings less risks. It is often the QR funding that gets projects to the stage where businesses will invest. So readers will not be surprised that university leaders want as much QR income as possible; hence, the drive to have the very best REF result.

Because of the human and physical resources that QR funds, those universities that perform well in the REF also attract research grants from other sources. These include research councils, major charities, the National Institute for Health Research (NIHR) and the European Union (EU). While some of these sources do not pay overheads or full economic costs, they still contribute approximately a further £2 billion per year to university research in the UK. Therefore, over the 6-year REF cycle, the sum allocated to UK universities from QR and other funding bodies is close to £24 billion per year.

The ultimate aim of the REF is to assess the quality of research in all the UK universities, in all disciplines [19]. It has a number of objectives. As stated above, the main one is to inform the selective allocation of public funding to universities for research. The Stern Report [20] identified others:

- To provide accountability for public investment in research and produce evidence of the benefits of this investment (impact)
- To provide benchmarking information and establish reputational yardsticks, for use within the HE sector and for public information
- To provide a rich evidence base to inform strategic decisions about national research priorities
- To create a strong performance incentive for universities and individual researchers
- To inform decisions on resource allocation by individual HEIs and other bodies

The REF assessment of the UK research is composed of three components: research outputs, research impact and research environment. Since the inception of research assessment exercises in the UK, outputs have been seen as the most important element. This was also the case in those other countries that assessed the quality of university research. However, in recent years, research impact has begun to eclipse outputs with regard to importance, at least in the UK. Steven Hill, Director of Research Policy for Research England, has argued that the justification for public funding of research rested primarily on the delivery of impact, which research assessments should therefore incentivise. He goes further by intimating that the weighting of impact assessment could be increased in future REF exercises [21].

1.3   The REF and Research Impact

As this book is being written in August 2020, the world is still in the grip of the Covid-19 pandemic. There is much discussion on when exactly the next REF will take place. The deadline for the submission was to be 27 November 2020. This has currently been extended to 31 March 2021. In some quarters, there are calls for the REF to be delayed further. Nonetheless, in this text, I will from time to time refer to REF2021; readers should take this as shorthand for the next REF.

A search of Digital Science's Dimensions database for scholarly articles published since the end of 2014 yields some 2000 papers that refer to the REF. The largest area of investigation of REF data has been impact case studies [22]. This provides insight into its importance. But even before impact was introduced into research assessments, there was a view that governments' financial support for research led to impact. Bush's [23] epochal report argued that publicly funded research would always pay off for society: excellent research would be followed by useful and practical applications. The 2014 REF helped evidence this by introducing research impact into the exercise.

However, it must be stressed that as a concept and movement, research impact is bigger than REF. At their best, universities are places where impact permeates all their activities from teaching to research and to academic enterprise. It should not be simply a task that university managers undertake every 6 years; rather it should be perceived as a public good and be culturally entrenched in all aspects of the institutions' culture, central to their sustainability.

The research impact agenda was driven by the perceptive questions being asked by politicians, treasury officials and others regarding what benefits accrued from the allocation of such large sums of public money. This was no surprise; at a time of economic hardship, governments require all forms of expenditure to be justified. The unspoken question was what impacts do 'state of the science' research infrastructure and research publications have for the UK economy and society? Furthermore, unless we can assess impact in some manner, it will be difficult to allocate public money for research in a way that maximises positive societal change.

The data from the 2014 REF have been retrospectively analysed by many investigators. One analysis was undertaken by Digital Science, a division of Macmillan Science and Education. It was partnered in this endeavour by Nature Publishing Group and the policy institute at King's College, London [22]. Using text mining and qualitative analysis techniques, they found widespread breadth and depth in research impact, supporting the extensive value that universities bring to wider society.

For instance, they found that over 80% of the research impact submitted included two or more 'field of research', illustrating the multidisciplinary nature of the research underpinning impact. Furthermore, the impacts were diverse and wide-ranging, with over 60 unique 'impact topics' identified. They reported that research impacts stemmed from research in a wide range of subject areas, with over 3,700 unique pathways from research to impact identified.

One finding that pleased the UK government was that research carried out in the UK had an impact in 195 countries—why is that important—it is every country in the world. Outside the UK, the most frequently identified countries were the United States, Australia, Canada, Germany and France. Therefore, the demonstration of research impact in the REF shows it to be a successful British export. This tells a story of strong

and diverse impact; albeit, there is some debate as to whether the benefits accrued more to foreign multinationals, economies and governments than to the UK [24].

In the REF, research excellence is judged on a 5-point scale (unclassified to 4 star). Impressively in the 2014 REF, 44% of the impacts were judged outstanding (4 star). A further 40% were judged very considerable impact (3 star); 13% were assessed as having considerable impact (2 star); 2% assessed as having recognised but modest impact (1 star); and 1% as having little or no impact (unclassified). Outstanding impacts were generated from research in all subjects. The results of the REF illustrate the many ways in which research has fuelled economic prosperity, influenced public policy and services, enhanced communities and civic society, enriched cultural life, improved health and well-being and tackled environmental challenges. In addition, outstanding impact was found across institutions with REF submissions of all sizes. These facts provide persuasive evidence for an austerity-focused UK Treasury that public research spending needs to be protected and increased.

An indication of how important research impact has become is demonstrated by it accounting for 25% of the total REF profile in the next exercise, up from 20% in the previous iteration. Research outputs will account for 65% and research environment 15%. Considering that the results of the exercise enable the allocation of over £10–12 billion between REF cycles, research impact accounts for a considerable percentage of that sum. The funding for this could be substantial for a university. Indeed, it has been reported by Dunleavy [25] that a single case study could be worth as much as £720,000 to a university over the 5-year REF period. It is important to note that universities also have to show in the research environment template how impact was enabled from their research activities; this adds a further sum of impact related income to universities' coffers.

Research impact is defined by Research England [19] as *an effect on, change or benefit to the economy, society, culture, public policy or services, health, the environment or quality of life*. As seen above, these effects, changes or benefits can occur both within the UK and overseas and can relate to the three 'Ps':

- *Processes*: the activity, attitude, awareness, behaviour, capacity, policy, opportunity, performance, practice or understanding
- *People*: an audience, families, beneficiary, community, constituency or individuals
- *Places*: any organisation or geographic location whether locally, regionally, nationally or internationally

So, for researchers, impacts can take many forms. These include impacts on health and welfare; impacts on society, culture and creativity; impacts on the economy; impacts on commerce; impacts on public policy and services; impacts on production; impacts on practitioners and services; impacts on the environment and impacts on international development.

1.4 Positive Views of Research Impact in the REF

Rand Europe [26] carried out an examination and analysis on the inclusion of research impact in the 2014 REF. The conclusion was that it was a success and both universities and expert panel members were supportive of its continued use in future assessment exercises. Both the big research-intensive universities and the smaller, specialist institutions performed well. Fears that trying to measure cultural, economic and societal impacts would lead to an overzealous pursuit of impact to the detriment of research were mostly unfounded.

From personal experience in the REF2014, I can vouch for this. A standard part of life for the academic members of the expert panels is the perpetual peer review of manuscripts for publication. Therefore, the assessment of outputs in the REF was not a novel experience for them. In contrast, they enjoyed the assessment of impact case studies. These were short interesting and read-

able descriptions of how research made a difference to society, the economy, health, etc. This was welcomed as a novel experience by expert panel assessors and a pleasant distraction from the assessment of numerous academic papers.

The REF also enabled researchers who were already engaging with research end-users and delivering positive impacts to have these outcomes formally recognised within a national assessment exercise and get rewarded for doing so. Other countries noted this and watched the inclusion of research impact in the REF with great interest. Many are already planning to assess impact as part of their future research assessment exercises. As in the UK, these governments believe it is not unreasonable to ask those whose research work is being undertaken at public expense to account for and provide some evidence of their activities and outcomes. Incidentally, the pilot for Excellence in Research for Australia (ERA) attempted to assess impact, but this did not find its way into the initial research exercise [27]. This has changed in a more recent iteration of the ERA and will be discussed later in Chap. 9.

1.5 Research Impact: Its Reach and Significance

In the REF, the expert panel assessors must judge the reach and significance of research impact. Here reach does not refer to geographic spread. Rather, it means the *extent and/or diversity of the beneficiaries of the impact*, as relevant to the nature of the impact [19]. In other words, what is the potential 'customer base' and how many are being impacted upon. This number of beneficiaries could be very small as in a cure for a very rare illness. Furthermore, local impact is not, by definition, inferior to international impact but is treated similarly in its assessment and rating. Therefore, an impact located within one region of the UK might be judged as 'outstanding' (graded as 4 star) or 'very considerable' (graded as 3 star). Equally, an impact located across several countries might not be judged as 'outstanding' or 'very considerable'. According to Grant and Hewlett [28], a reasonable estimate is that just under 20% of impact submitted to REF 2014 demonstrated local research impact.

The *significance* of a research impact focuses on the *intensity of the influence* or degree to which the impact has enabled, enriched, influenced, informed or changed the performance, policies, practices, products, services, understanding, awareness or well-being of the beneficiaries [19]. Questions we could ask here include: has the uptake and implementation of the research results cured a disease, extended lifespan, eliminated some harm, enhanced quality of life, produced a new effective healthcare drug or product?

It is possible for an impact case study to be outstanding with regard to significance but with little or no reach or vice versa. To illustrate this, research findings from a medical study may have excellent dissemination, achieved good publicity in the media and at conferences, leading many people to be aware of their existence. In this instance, its reach may be categorised as outstanding. However, in terms of significance, the intensity and the influence of the research may be modest or low. To gain a grasp of research impact, one must ask what benefit or change resulted from the outstanding reach? Similarly, a research study on hospital-acquired infection in a local health trust may have outstanding significance for that hospital, but the reach is modest. So, reach or significance in isolation is not sufficient to claim research impact.

In assessing the impact described within a case study, the REF expert panel will form an overall combined view about its 'reach and significance'. In other words, they will be taken as a whole, rather than assessed separately. Based on this, the expert panel assessors will allocate a star rating for quality (see Table 1.1).

For health research, impact could relate to improved health or welfare outcomes, enhanced professional standards, ethics, guidelines or training, improved quality, accessibility or efficiency of a public service or changes in professional practice or the development of a new incontinence product. It is not unreasonable to think that identifying research impact for the health professions should be straightforward. After all, they are applied disciplines, and it should be possible to trace how the findings of research studies have changed practice, product or policy.

Table 1.1 The REF quality ratings for impact case studies [19]

4 star	Outstanding impacts in terms of their reach and significance
3 star	Very considerable impacts in terms of their reach and significance
2 star	Considerable impacts in terms of their reach and significance
1 star	Recognised but modest impacts in terms of their reach and significance
Unclassified	The impact is of little or no reach and significance; or the impact was not eligible; or the impact was not underpinned by excellent research produced by the submitted unit

Reflection Point 1.4 Examples of Research Impact

Consider possible answers to the questions posed in Table 1.2.

I will attempt to answer these questions, but before I do, readers should remember three key messages:

- Impact must have such a strong link to underpinning research to such an extent that without the research, the impact would not have happened.
- Dissemination is not impact.
- To have impact, something must change, there should be some benefit.

Table 1.2 Questions to consider with regard to Research Impact

- Is writing a bestselling book impact?
- Is speaking about your research findings at a conference, on radio or on television impact?
- Is providing a continuing professional education (CPD) course to the staff of a private nursing home impact?
- Is showing that a particular procedure should no longer be undertaken impact?

Take the question about the bestselling book. OK, so the publisher's profits may have been enhanced or the writer's profile may have been improved but did anything really change as a result of people buying or reading the book and if so, how is this evidenced? Think here of 'reach' and 'significance'. Due to thousands of people buying it, the bestselling book may have an outstanding reach, but what was the significance of this? Did people read the book? I am reminded here of James Joyce's Ulysses, a novel that is famous for people starting it but not finishing it. But if people did read the bestseller, did they behave differently or think differently as a result of reading it?

The same analysis applies to the second question: How do you know if anything has changed because research findings were shared through conferences or through the media? What is the evidence that there were some benefits?

Similarly, how do you know if there has been any benefit from running a CPD course in a private nursing home? Did the home owners simply meet their in-house training requirements or did the nursing home staff simply include this in their regulatory body's re-registration exercise? Perhaps thinking or behaviour did not change.

Providing evidence of the reach and significance of research impact is a crucial but difficult task. So, if you surveyed a sample of your readers, viewers or listeners and found that they had changed their practice as a result of your research and this had a positive impact on patients, this is a good start to develop your evidence base for impact.

What if a large nursing home company changed its processes, policies or practices as a result of your research-led CPD course and this improved the quality of life and health and well-being of their residents? This too would provide the basis for reach and significance.

So far, most of the examples of impact used were positive. In other words, the research results started the initiation of a new intervention or practice that had positive results. However, negative examples are also relevant where research has led to something being stopped rather than started.

From time to time, research findings allow us to stop some long-established ritualistic practices and make care and treatment safer for patients. No reasonable person would dispute the benefit of this, and therefore, this is another example of research impact that could have outstanding reach and significance. For example, personalised medicine research that showed the ineffectiveness of anti-hypertensive medication for populations with a specific genome could be an example of outstanding reach and significance due to stopping prescribing practices for this cohort. Therefore, outstanding (4 star) research impact can include the reduction or prevention of harm, risk, cost or other negative effects.

1.6   The REF Expert Panels

For the purposes of the REF, the different research subject areas in UK universities are designated as Units of Assessment (UoA). For the next exercise there are 34 of these and the REF assessment is undertaken by 34 corresponding expert panels, grouped under four main panels:

- Main Panel A: Medical and Life Sciences
- Main Panel B: Physical Sciences and Engineering
- Main Panel C: Social Sciences
- Main Panel D: Arts and Humanities

Each main panel comprises a chair, international members, impact assessor members, the REF team administrators and the chairs of the expert panels. While the structures and processes have similiarities across all four main panels, I will use Main Panel A, the Medical and Life Sciences Panel as an exemplar (MPA). It is composed of six expert subpanels reflecting distinct UoAs: UoA1 (Clinical Medicine), UoA2, (Public Health, Health Services and Primary Care), UoA3 (Allied Health Professions, Dentistry, Nursing and Pharmacy), UoA4 (Psychology, Psychiatry and Neuroscience), UoA5 (Biological Sciences) and UoA6 (Agriculture, Veterinary and Food Science). For each of these subpanels, there will be approximately 20–50 members. Some will be full members; some will be output assessors and some will be impact assessors.

The full members tend to be senior academics, mostly professors, whose role is to assess the outputs (mainly journal papers in MPA and MPB), impact case studies and research environment templates submitted to the REF by the UK universities. Reflected in their title, output assessors will only review the quality of outputs and have no role in the assessment of research impact or the research environment. Impact assessors will mainly focus on reviewing the impact case studies but may have a role in assessing those elements of the environment that deal with the enabling of research impact.

These expert panel members have to be nominated by a range of organisations and groups; they cannot be selected by universities. From a long list of nominees, panel members are selected for their specific expertise. Care is taken to ensure that there are not too many from the same university, that all countries in the UK are represented

and that there is equity with regard to gender and race. Conflicts of interest are also taken into account. Once these criteria have been followed, the four funding bodies have to approve and sign off the successful appointees.

1.7   Summary

This chapter represented a taster for research impact. Readers will have learned that this is not some passing fad; rather, it will increase in importance. This is driven by the fervent desire to demonstrate to taxpayers and charitable donors that their investments are bringing benefits to the economy, culture, society and health care. An overview of the REF was presented and how expert panel assessors are selected, appointed and undertake their work. Questions were posed on various scenarios, and the importance of reach and significance for each was explored. This sets the scene for Chap. 2, which will deal with the research impact case study.

References

1. Gray, GT. Gray, SW. Customer retention in sports organization marketing: examining the impact of team identification and satisfaction with team performance. Int. J. Consum. 2012. https://doi.org/10.1111/j.1470-6431.2011.00999.x.
2. Cambridge Dictionary. Impact. Cambridge: Cambridge University Press; 2020. https://dictionary.cambridge.org/.
3. Collins. Business dictionaries – pocket business English dictionary. London: Collins; 2012. ISBN: 978-0-00-745420-4. https://collins.co.uk/pages/about.
4. Banzi R, Moja L, Pistotti V, Facchinni A, Liberati A. Conceptual frameworks and empirical approaches used to assess the impact of health research: an overview of reviews. Health Res Policy Syst. 2011;9:26. https://doi.org/10.1186/1478-4505-9-26. PMCID: PMC3141787.
5. UKRI. Research excellence framework. Swindon: United Kingdom Research and Innovation; 2020. https://re.ukri.org/research/research-excellence-framework-ref/.
6. Nightingale F. Notes on nursing; what it is, and what it is not. D. Appleton and Company: New York, NY; 1860.

7. Bacon F. Selected philosophical works. Indianapolis, IN: Hackett Pub; 1999. ISBN 0-87220-470-7. OCLC 41211508.

8. United Nations. Sustainability development goals 2030. New York, NY: United Nations; 2015. https://www.un.org/sustainabledevelopment/sustainable-development-goals/.

9. Block WH. Justus Freiherr Von Liebig. Encyclopaedia Britannica; 2020. https://www.britannica.com/biography/Justus-Freiherr-von-Liebig.

10. EHEA. The Magna Charta Universitatum. Bologna: EHEA; 1988. http://www.ehea.info/cid101830/magna-charta.html.

11. Dearing R. The Dearing report: higher education in the learning society. London: Her Majesty's Stationery Office; 1997. http://www.educationengland.org.uk/documents/dearing1997/dearing1997.html. Accessed Mar 2020.

12. OECD. Education. Paris: Organization for Economic Co-operation and Development; 2020. https://www.oecd.org/education/.

13. Hamdullahpur F. How to forge stronger ties between universities and industry. The Times Higher Education; 2017. https://www.timeshighereducation.com/blog/how-forge-stronger-ties-between-universities-and-industry.

14. Baker S. Do university excellence initiatives work? The Times Higher Education; 2020. https://www.timeshighereducation.com/features/do-university-excellence-initiatives-work.

15. UK Parliament. The Haldane principle. London: House of Commons; 2009. https://publications.parliament.uk/pa/cm200809/cmselect/cmdius/168/16807.htm.

16. Penfield T, Baker MJ, Scoble R, Wykes MC. Assessment, evaluations, and definitions of research impact: a review. Res Eval. 2014;23(1):21–32. https://doi.org/10.1093/reseval/rvt021.

17. Carr D. Maximising the value of research outputs: Wellcome's perspective. London: Wellcome; 2018. https://www.belmontforum.org/wp-content/uploads/2019/10/Carr-WellcomeTrust_OpenSci.pdf.

18. Department for Business; Energy; Industrial Strategy. Building on success and learning from experience an independent review of the research excellence framework. London: Department for Business, Energy & Industrial Strategy; 2016.

19. Research England. The research excellence framework. Swindon: Research England; 2020. https://re.ukri.org/research/research-excellence-framework-ref/.

20. Stern N. Building on success and learning from experience an independent review of the research excellence framework. London: Department of Business, Energy and Industrial Strategy; 2016. https://assets.publishing.service.gov.uk/government/uploads/system/uploads/attachment_data/file/541338/ind-16-9-ref-stern-review.pdf.

21. Hill S. Assessing (for) impact: future assessment of the societal impact of research. London: Palgrave Communications; 2016. https://doi.org/10.1057/palcomms.2016.73.

22. Digital Science. The societal and economic impacts of academic research international perspectives on good practice and managing evidence; 2016. https://www.digital-science.com/resources/digital-research-reports/digital-research-report-societal-economic--impacts-academic-research/.

23. Bush V. Science: the endless frontier, a report to president Truman outlining his proposal for post-war U.S. science and technology policy. Washington, DC: United States Government Printing Office; 1945.

24. Khazragui H. Measuring the benefits of university research: impact and the REF in the UK. Res Eval. 2014;24(1):51–62. https://doi.org/10.1093/reseval/rvu028.

25. Dunleavy P. 'REF advice note 1. Understanding HEFCE's definition of impact', LSE impact of social sciences blog; 2012. http://blogs.lse.ac.uk/impactofsocialsciences/2012/10/22/dunleavy-ref-advice-1/. Accessed 7 Jun 2020.

26. Rand Europe. Lessons from EU Research Funding (1998-2013). Published in: EU Law and Publications. https://doi.org/10.2777/667857. Posted on RAND.org on December 15, 2017. https://www.rand.org/pubs/external_publications/EP67423.html.

27. McKenna HP, Daly J, Davidson P, Duffield C, Jackson D. RAE and ERA – spot the difference. Int. J. Nurs. 2012;49(4):375–77.

28. Grant J, Hewlett K. Putting impact in its place. Research Fortnight. 2019. https://www.researchprofessional.com/0/rr/news/uk/views-of-the-uk/2019/9/Putting-impact-in-itsplace.html?utm_medium=email&utm_source=rpMailing&utm_campaign=researchFortnightNews_2019-09-04#sthash.DQR1zNmy.dpuf.

Research Impact: Drafting Case Studies

2

Genius is in the idea. Impact, however, comes from action.
Simon Sinek [1]

2.1   Introduction

In the Research Excellence Framework (REF), 'Academic Impact' is assessed in the review of research outputs [2]. This includes the significance, rigour and originality of the outputs. However, research impact or what some people refer to as societal impact is judged by the assessment of five-page impact case studies (ICS). These will be analysed in detail below. They are based on the cause and effect principle—what is referred to as the 'underpinning research' triggered the impact. In other words, the findings from the supporting research made a distinct and material contribution to social, economic, health or cultural effect, change or benefit.

In the 2021 REF, the definition of research impact was broadened since its introduction in the previous iteration in 2014. This was recommended by Sir Nicholas Stern, who chaired a REF Evaluation Committee [3]. The Committee made it clear that impact case studies should not be narrowly interpreted and need not solely focus on socio-economic impacts. Rather, case studies should take a wide view of impact, including government policy, public engagement and understanding, cultural life, university curricula and pedagogy. The Committee wanted REF to capture, in a more meaningful way, the multiple and diverse pathways and mechanisms through which impact arises. This led to enhanced clarity and a broadening in the description of underpinning research from a reliance on outputs in REF 2014 to 'bodies of work' in REF 2021.

One example of this is the impact on teaching. Previously, an impact case study on teaching could only be submitted in the REF if the effect, benefit or change was external to the submitting university. In other words, an impact case study would get an unclassified rating if the research carried out in University A only had an impact on teaching and learning in University A. This was changed following the Stern recommendations where the impact on teaching *within* (and beyond) a submitting university is now eligible. However, it is a challenge (though not impossible) to come up with examples of such impacts where the reach and significance would be judged as outstanding.

In the UK, teaching excellence within universities is rewarded in a parallel exercise called the Teaching Excellence Framework [4]. It would be wrong for a university to get rewarded twice for the same impact. Therefore, expert panel members might expect that impact on teaching within the submitting university to convincingly form a component of a wider case study that also includes impacts beyond the institution.

2.2   The REF Impact Case Study Template

2.2.1   Stylistic Issues

Drafting impact case studies is more of an art than a science. A reader without specialist knowledge should be able to understand the narrative. It is important to write them in understandable English using an active authorship style with concise sentences rather than complicated scientific jargon. Acronyms should be avoided whenever possible. (*Note*: In the UK, it may be the case that a university in Wales could submit an impact case study written in Welsh.)

In the 2014 REF, some universities hired journalists to draft their impact case studies or had their communications or press office edit them for readability. This may not have been uniformly successful as it may lead the researchers to become concerned that their work was being 'oversold'. Ebullient re-writes in 'marketing speak' may not go down well with expert panel assessors. They may interpret a journalistic style as a dumbing down or a deliberate unnecessary oversimplification of the science. As a result, the impact case study may receive a lower quality rating. Readers should not forget that the academic and impact assessors on the expert panels are quite proficient in their respective topic areas. Accepting this, the services of a knowledgably and sensible science writer, working alongside the researchers, may make a positive difference to readability and understanding.

Universities may include URLs in the impact case studies but only for the purpose of verifying claims made. However, readers should note that expert panel assessors will not follow URLs to access additional evidence or information. Case studies should include sufficiently clear and detailed information to enable assessors to make judgements based on the information it contains, without making inferences, gathering additional material, following up references or relying on assessors' prior knowledge. All the materials required to make a judgement should be included in the case study template, and no further reading should be required. The trick is to make it easy for the assessors and provide them with a clear and coherent narrative supported by verifiable evidence and indicators.

Completed impact case study templates may include formatting (bold or underlined text, headings, lists and so on), tables and non-text content, so long as the guidance is followed on the maximum page limit, on minimum font size, on line spacing and on margin widths.

While there are indicative number of words for the various sections, there is some flexibility. Each completed case study will be limited to five pages in length, including all references. Table 2.1 lists the fields that are required to enable submitting UoAs to provide key information about a case study's eligibility. The page limit excludes the personal details of the corroborating sources listed in Section M in Table 2.1. A note of caution: those drafting the case studies should be careful not to extend some sections to the detriment of others.

In addition to Sections A–M, submitting UoAs are required to complete, where applicable, additional contextual data fields. This information

Table 2.1 The REF Impact Case Study template

A. The name of the submitting university
B. The Unit of Assessment where the impact case study applies
C. The period when the underpinning research was undertaken
D. The names and roles of staff conducting the underpinning research from the submitting unit
E. The period when staff involved in the underpinning research were employed by the submitting university
F. The period when the claimed impact occurred
G. Whether the case study is a continued case study
H. The title of the case study
I. A summary of the research impact in 100 words
J. A description of the research underpinning the impact (500 words)
K. References to the research (up to six)
L. Details of the research impact (700 words)
M. Sources to corroborate the research impact (up to ten sources)

will enable research funders to track and evaluate the impact of their funding. It will also aid the use and analysis of case studies following the end of the exercise. These details will not be provided to the expert panel assessors; rather, they will be collected in a separate form and will not form part of the five-page limit:

- Name(s) of funder(s)
- Global Research Identifier of funder(s): https://www.grid.ac/
- Name(s) of funding programme(s)
- Grant number(s)
- Amount of grant (in GBP (Sterling))
- ORCID for each named researcher, where held
- Name(s) of formal partner(s)
- Country/countries where the impact occurred

Because this contextual information is not provided to expert panels nor will it form part of the assessment process, I will focus solely on the sections in Table 2.1.

A. The Name of the Submitting University

There are three points to make here. First, the submitting institution may not be a university; it could be a college or a research foundation. For instance, the Institute of Cancer Research, the Courtauld Institute of Art and the Royal College of Music make REF submissions. Second, occasionally a university takes over a research centre from another institution. In this case, the university can return impact case studies from underpinning research that was conducted in the research centre before it became part of the submitting university, as long as it had a distinct and material contrition to the impact claimed. This has to be approved by the relevant UK funding body. Third, there are also instances where two or more universities merge for the purposes of REF and they make a single joint submission.

Common Misunderstanding in This Section
Where two or more universities are submitting a joint REF return, all universities have an equivalent lead role in the process.

This Is Incorrect
For administrative purposes, one university needs to be identified as the lead institution in terms of management and data security of a joint submission. Impact case studies should be submitted by the Lead University on behalf of all the other universities in the joint submission.

B. The Unit of Assessment Where the Impact Case Study Applies

Here too, more than one university may merge their UoAs into a single REF return, and the same principle applies as outlined in the previous section. It is also worth remembering that as long as the underpinning research is within the scope of the UoA in which the case study is submitted, it may be returned in a different UoA from the individuals who conducted the underpinning research. This is because individual researchers may undertake research across multiple disciplines over time, and it is accepted that UoA boundaries are permeable.

Common Misunderstanding in This Section
An impact case study in a submitting university can only relate to one UoA.

This Is Incorrect
All UoAs that conducted elements of the research, that made a material and distinct contribution to the impact, can submit an impact case study in the REF return. Each must acknowledge the input of the researchers in the other UoAs.

C. The Period When the Underpinning Research Was Undertaken

The underpinning research must have occurred during a specified 20-year period. For REF 2021, the timeframe is between 1 January 2000 and 31 December 2020. Where the appearance of the final version of an underpinning output has been delayed due to Covid-19, and is not in the public domain by the 31 December 2020, the submitting institution should return the final form by the 31 March 2021. This is for exceptional cases and the fact that it is a delayed output should be clearly identified.

Common Misunderstanding in This Section
The underpinning research has to have been conducted after 1 January 2000.

This Is Incorrect
In some cases, the underpinning research started before 1 January 2000 but continued, and the published outputs came into the public domain after that date.

D. The Names and Roles of Staff Conducting the Underpinning Research from the Submitting UoA

This section requires details of the job titles of staff and their roles at the time when the underpinning research was conducted. This is to validate that the staff were active researchers in the submitting UoA when the underpinning research was undertaken (1 January 2000 to 31 December 2020; see proviso above). However, there may be rare occasions when this is not the case. For example, the researchers conducted the study shortly before 1 January 2000. In this case, the publications from that study might only appear in the public domain on or after 1 January 2000, and the researcher(s) had left the submitting university in the time period between these two points.

Common Misunderstandings in This Section
(a) The underpinning research has to have been conducted by staff who had their publications submitted in the 'Outputs' component of the REF.

(b) The research underpinning the impact should have been done by a single researcher.
(c) The researchers conducting the study or the university where the research was conducted have to have been involved in generating the impact.

These Are All Incorrect
(a) It is stated above that the REF is composed of three components, Research Outputs, Research Impact and Research Environment, each of which are assessed separately. It is possible that the researchers whose publications underpinned the impact case study did not submit these for assessment in the output component of the REF.
(b) This may be the case in some disciplines, but is not a requirement in any. In most of the science, technology and engineering disciplines, impact case studies are often the result of projects undertaken by several researchers working in interdisciplinary teams.
(c) Traditionally, researchers and universities were not expected to have been involved actively in developing impact from their studies. This is still the case but may change in future assessment exercises as a result of the more proactive approach that researchers take in identifying pathways to impact (see the Introduction in Chap. 1).

E. The Period When Staff Involved in the Underpinning Research Were Employed by the Submitting University

The justification for these details is that research impact is non-portable. The submitting university has the ownership of the research impact, and it cannot be retained by researchers who move to employment in other institutions.

Therefore, if the researcher or an entire research team moved to another university after the research was complete, they cannot bring the research impact with them. In essence, universities cannot 'buy in' research impact. Attempting to claim research impact by a submitting university UoA when the underpinning research was not conducted there would result in an unclassified grade for that case study—not a good outcome.

However, researchers often move to a different institution before the related outputs of the underpinning research are in the public domain. In such a case, the submitting university must make clear that the underpinning research was carried out when the researcher was at their institution. They must also evidence that it made a distinct and material contribution to the impact claimed. Similarly, it is possible that the research outputs came into the public domain when the researchers were at the submitting university but the underpinning research had been conducted at the researcher(s)' previous place of employment. In this case, if the submitting university attempts to claim the impact, it would obtain an unclassified rating.

There are other complexities when researchers change employment during a REF cycle. It is given that the best impact case studies tend to be written by the researchers who conducted the research. However, if the researcher(s) has moved to another university, it is very difficult to get them to tell their impact 'story' for their previous employer, especially since their research impact is non-portable. Their reason for moving universities may also affect their willingness to assist a previous employer.

Common Misunderstandings in This Section
(a) Impacts from projects conducted by research students can be submitted by them in REF.
(b) The researchers who conducted the research must be employed by the submitting university.

These Are All Incorrect
(a) Research undertaken solely by research students is not considered as having been carried out by staff while working in the submitting university. Research students are not perceived within REF as being 'independent researchers'.
(b) Academic staff who conducted the underpinning research may not be employed by the submitting university; as outlined above, they may have obtained employment in another university. It is also legitimate for Category C staff to have conducted the underpinning research. These are individuals who are not on the payroll of the university, but most of their research activities are clearly focused in the submitting university. For example, they may be employed by the NHS, a Research Council unit, a charity or other organisation. Furthermore, the researchers may have been unpaid staff or staff who have retired from the university but conducted the studies prior to their departure.

F. The Period When the Claimed Impact Occurred

Because of the hiatus caused by the Covid-19 pandemic, at the time of going to press, the research impact must occur between 1 August 2013 and 31 December 2020. This represents a 5-month extension from the previous advertised ending date. This has positive and negative implications. For the former, it means that research impacts relating to Covid-19 research may be included in the forthcoming REF. For the latter, it means that those research impacts that were negatively affected by Covid can be included. Examples of this include those public engagement events, sporting events or overseas research activities that were cancelled or postponed. An optional verifiable statement (max 100 words) may be provided to explain the Covid-19 disruption to impact activities. This may include an explanation of delays to planned events or the collection of key corroboration sources.

This may include impacts that started prior to 1 August 2013 but continued into the impact census period. Regardless, case studies will be assessed to ensure that the impact's reach and significance only occurred during the period 1 August 2013 to 31 December 2020. Any case studies submitted that claim impact prior to or after this census period will be awarded an unclassified score. Institutions should not consider it necessary to amend existing case studies to report up to the end of December 2020. The REF panels do not expect nor require that all case studies report up to this date. Those reporting to the previous deadline of 31 Jul 2020 will be assessed on an equal footing with those delayed due to Covid-19.

Common Misunderstanding in This Section
The underpinning research always has to have been conducted before the impact happens.

This Is Incorrect
The relationship between the underpinning research and the realisation of impact may not always follow a linear pathway. Impact can occur contemporaneously with the underpinning research, and it is possible that impact can occur before the research outputs, underpinning the research come into the public domain.

G. Whether the Case Study Is a Continued Case Study

The REF exercise takes place every 5–6 years. As has been outlined above, the last one was in 2014 and the next (depending on the outworkings of the Covid-19 pandemic) will be in 2021. The Stern Committee [3] recognised that

impact generation can be a lengthy ongoing process. Hence, case studies returned in one REF could evolve and be resubmitted in subsequent REFs. There were almost 7000 un-redacted case studies submitted in REF 2014. The question that arises is how many of these will have matured in some way and be submitted in REF 2021 as continued case studies? A definition of a continued case study is that it does not describe any new research having taken place that has made a distinct or material contribution since it was submitted in 2014 and the body of underpinning research is the same as described in the 2014 case study.

To explain this, I will use the example of climbing Mount Everest—you would agree that getting to base camp is an impact but moving on to the summit is a continued impact. Both have reach and significance. Getting to base camp could be a REF 2014 impact, whereas reaching the summit could be an impact in the next REF. The obvious question with this example is what would be the impact in the following REF? This poses another important question of how far along the pathway of benefit or change does something need to be for impact to be claimed?

Because they are continued case studies, by definition, one would expect that what is submitted in the next REF will have significant overlap with what was submitted in REF 2014. In other words, the impact types and beneficiaries are broadly the same as described in the 2014 case study. Compared to the other three main panels, Main Panel A has a slightly different view about continued case studies. It recognises the long lead-in time and evolution of impact and so expects to see continued case studies being submitted. Nonetheless, it encourages the submission of new case studies to show the vitality and vibrancy of healthcare research.

For REF 2014, the period for the underpinning research was 1 January 1993 to 31 December 2013. As can be seen above, this overlaps by 14 years with the period for underpinning research in the next REF (1 January 2000 to 31 December 2020). This means that some or all of the underpinning research outputs could be included in both the exercises. This overlap makes continued case studies possible as the same research outputs can be used twice.

By definition, a new impact case study is one where new research was conducted since the 2014 REF that has made a distinct and material contribution to the impact, and/or the impact types or beneficiaries have changed. Hence, for a new impact case study, assessors would expect to see that some or all of the outputs reflecting the underpinning research were in the public domain after 31 December 2013 and/or that new beneficiaries have benefited and/or a new impact occurred. The and/or is important here as this shows that a new impact case study may not have new research conducted since 2014, but the original underpinning research has impacted upon new groups or professions or organisations. For instance, a REF 2014 impact case study concerning community dentistry may in the next REF benefit general practitioners. Even though no more research was undertaken, this is a new impact case study, rather than a continued one. Similarly, a new impact may have arisen; for example, a new economic impact rather than the previous health or social or cultural one.

Submitting units are expected to flag continued case studies. This information will be made available to subpanels and will be used by the funding bodies in post-assessment evaluations. Irrespective of whether an impact is continuing or not, the key question for the assessors will be whether it stands up as a case study in its own right.

Common Misunderstanding in This Section
(a) A continued impact case study always needs new research evidence to underpin it since its previous REF submission.
(b) Researchers who moved to another university and whose research activities have continued can count the impact from their previous and current institutions.

These Are Incorrect
(a) If there was new underpinning research, then this would be a new impact case study, not a continuing one.
(b) Researchers can only claim the impact from the point at which they conducted investigations in their current university. While any impact prior to that point may be described in the case study as background, it can only be claimed by the researchers' previous university.

H. The Title of the Case Study

It is often the case that the title of an impact case study is the first thing an assessor reads but the last thing a university researcher writes. The title should be snappy, informative, compelling and memorable. It might be a good idea to begin it with a verb such as 'Transforming treatment for…' or 'Improving care in…'or 'Producing a novel intervention…', etc. In essence, the title should be concise and precise, reflecting the impact that is being claimed. For example, an impact case describing a clinical guideline for cardiac rehabilitation entitled 'Shoot for goal' is not reflective enough of the impact. Furthermore, interested parties looking for cardiac rehabilitation impact would not identify this impact case study in a searchable data base.

Common Misunderstanding in This Section
The title needs to be a catchy sound bite.

This Is Incorrect
The title should be a brief description of the impact being claimed.

I. The Summary of the Impact

The REF assessors get their first impressions of the impact in this section, and it is a truism that first impressions are lasting. The summary of the impact needs to be a clear succinct explanation of the impact that has resulted from the underpinning research. It is not a summary of the entire case study. There is no need to mention the underpinning research, but this may be difficult, depending on the impact. It is helpful if the gaps that the research addressed are identified and a good idea to highlight briefly how the impact claimed had reach and significance. The following research impact summary is from a 4 star impact case study submitted by the University of Southampton in the 2014 REF.

There are currently 2 million cancer survivors in the UK. This is predicted to become 6 million by 2050—by which time more than 50% of the UK population are expected to have experienced a cancer diagnosis. Our research and expertise have been central to the creation of the Department of Health's National Cancer Survivorship Initiative (NCSI) and framing policy more widely to respond to this challenge. It has provided evidence of the wide-ranging impact of the disease following cancer treatment and has led to new models of cancer aftercare being implemented across the UK and internationally.

https://impact.ref.ac.uk/casestudies/CaseStudy.aspx?Id=43851

In this summary, readers will note the absence of jargon and the use of plain English. The research problem is described in the first sentence. This is followed by the benefit and change that the research has achieved. The underpinning research is not described. The last sentence also intimates reach and significance.

> **Common Misunderstanding in This Section**
> That the summary is a brief overview of the entire case study.

> **This Is Incorrect**
> It should only focus on a brief description of the impact.

J. Research Underpinning the Impact

This section has an allocated maximum length of 500 words. This is where the expert panel assessors seek convincing evidence that the research undertaken at the submitting university led to the impact that is being claimed. In other words, it was this research that made the difference. The impact may be the result of a body of research produced over a number of years or may be the result of a single project. While you may not include it in this section, the counterfactual is worth considering; what would have happened had the research not been conducted. If the answer is that the impact would not have happened, then the link between the underpinning research and the impact is strong.

If possible, it is a good idea to write the impact case study indicating that the impact had been planned when the research was planned. After REF 2014, feedback from Main Panel A indicated that the most convincing case studies are those that made it clear that the pathway to impact was a specific objective from the outset and that it had been achieved. This works well with applied research, but the case is not as compelling for curiosity-driven blue skies research. For example, a social scientist may plan a research project around the objective of changing policy, whereas a mathematician would be less able to make a persuasive case that the impact was planned from the beginning. This means that making the case for impact being planned from the outset is specific to different research designs, methodologies and disciplines.

Following the Stern Report [3], it was recommended that the allusion to underpinning research was too traditional and too narrow a view of what could create impact. Rather, it was suggested that there should be a broadening of the sources and types of impacts allowed, so that case studies could be linked to a body of work and a broad range of research. While this broadening is welcome, in the context of health science research, the term 'accompanying research' instead of 'underpinning research' might be better as this is less linear in its implications. Nonetheless, because it is the most common parlance, the latter term will be used in this textbook.

In the description of the underpinning research, references to outputs should be included that embody the research and provide evidence of its quality. This can be done by signifying a reference in this section as R1, R2, R3, etc., and in the next section, the actual references will be included with these identifiers. If possible, this section should refer to references that will enable the expert panel assessors to be confident that the 2 star threshold has been met.

The research aims, objectives or research questions should be briefly described as should the methodology and findings. This gives the expert panel assessors insight into the work that underpinned the impact and how, when and by whom it was conducted. Furthermore, there should be a brief explanation of what is original or distinctive about the research insights that contributed to the impact.

The research underpinning the impact may have been part of a larger body of work involving researchers from other UoAs in the same or in different universities. In this instance, the case study should specify the particular contribution of the researchers in the submitted UoA, while acknowledging the key research contributions from researchers in the other UoAs.

To illustrate the above, readers should undertake the following exercise on a 4 star impact case study from the University of Bristol. Follow the web link below and check if the university adhered to these guidelines when they described the research that led to improving care for children born with cleft lip and palate in the UK and beyond.

https://impact.ref.ac.uk/casestudies/CaseStudy.aspx?Id=40173

Common Misunderstanding in This Section
(a) The underpinning research should be funded.
(b) Universities should not use the same body of research to underpin more than one impact case study.

These Are Incorrect
(a) In many instances, the underpinning research is not funded (see Fig 8.6, Chap. 8).
(b) Universities can use the same body of research for different impact case studies. However, there is a danger of salami slicing and the dilution of reach and significance for the different impacts described.

K. The References to the Research

In this section, references to key outputs from the research described in the previous section and evidence about the quality of the research are provided. As alluded to in the previous section, it is important to show that the research underpinning the impact is of at least 2 star quality. This is defined as *quality that is recognised nationally in terms of originality, significance and rigour.* The outputs referenced here should be able to convince the expert panel assessors that the research achieved or exceeded this level of quality.

Each impact case study can have up to six published references that emanated from the underpinning research. While these can be reports, portfolios and other types of outputs, in health-related UoAs, they tend to be published papers. The references will also help flag for the assessors that the reported research entered the public domain between 1 January 2000 and 31 December 2020 (See C above for Covid-19 related delays).

The types of outputs listed in this section vary. In the 2014 REF, 11,822 journal papers (91.7%) were used as references for the underpinning research submitted to Main Panel A. There were also 274 books or book chapters (2.1%), 150 conference proceedings (1.2%) and 631 (4.9%) other sources such as research reports. The types of outputs need not be limited to printed academic work. In fact, those submitted to the other main panels may include, but are not limited to, new materials, devices, images, artefacts, products and buildings; confidential or technical reports;

intellectual property, whether in patents or other forms; performances, exhibits or events; work published in non-print media. The expert panel assessors will consider all forms of output referencing the underpinning research equitably with no one type being preferred over another. While it is often disputed by researchers, there is no hierarchy of output types.

Each output included in this section of the impact case study should include the following: the author(s), title, year of publication, type of output and other relevant details to identify the output (e.g. journal title, issue number, page number). In addition, to link it to the preceding and succeeding sections, each output can be designated R1, R2, R3, etc. A further issue worth remembering is that the outputs underpinning the research impact may not have been authored or created by full-time members of staff in the submitting university (see Section E above).

While it is not necessarily the case, the output may also have been submitted in the output category of REF. There is some overlap between the two categories. In total, there are 120,784 journal papers in the REF 2014 database of submitted research outputs and 11,822 journal papers among the case study references. Of these, 5703 papers feature in both [5]. The submitting UoAs must have been certain that these were 3 or 4 star quality. If they were 2 star quality, they would not attract any QR money; only 3 and 4 star outputs attract funding. It is interesting to reflect here that research impact underpinned by 2 star outputs could attract significant QR funding for the submitting university, but the same outputs would not reach the threshold to receive QR funding if submitted through the research output component of REF.

There should also be details on how the assessors can access the outputs, if required. This can be through a Digital Object Identifier (DoI), a hard copy or through a web link. For some expert panels, the outputs are stored in a central warehouse. These can be paintings, sculptures, books or artefacts. In other instances, the output will be supplied on request by the submitting university.

There is space in the template for a short description of each output. This should not include citation indices or impact factors of journals. For the former, expert panel assessors will be supplied with citation indices by Clarivate Analytics. For the latter, Research England, who manage the REF for the UK government, has signed up the San Francisco Declaration of Research Assessment [6]. This prohibits the use of journal impact factors for the assessment of research quality.

Those who draft impact case studies should remember that the expert panel assessors will have to read and assess several hundred publications in the research output category of REF. When it comes to assessing impact case studies, they will be presented with up to another six outputs to assess. They will not expect each referenced item to meet the 2 star threshold, but will wish to be satisfied that the research as a whole was of at least this quality. Where assessors identify at least one output of 2 star quality or higher, and this is a key output underpinning the impact, this will normally be sufficient to demonstrate that the underpinning research meets the quality threshold.

Submitting universities should make it easy for the expert panel assessors. Where available, they can include proxies in the form of prizes, prestigious grants, awards, etc. indicative of 2 star quality and above. This will provide confidence to the assessors that the outputs are at least 2 star quality. Furthermore, when possible, the best outputs should be placed at the start of the list of six.

Assuming that the expert panel assessors are convinced that the research was of at least 2 star quality, was conducted at the submitting university and made a material contribution to the impact, then the threshold is met. These outputs will play no further role in the assessment, and the expert panel assessors will move onto the impact itself. It is worth noting that 11% of audit queries in REF 2014 related to the underpinning research and 25% of these were subsequently rated as unclassified [7].

While the heading for this section explicitly focuses on references, brief details of research grants should also be included. Particulars should comprise who the grant was awarded to, the grant title, the sponsor, the period of the grant (with dates) and the value of the grant.

Common Misunderstandings in This Section

(a) The underpinning research output must be in published journal articles.

(b) If the output has the submitting university's address on it, then the research was conducted there.

(c) The references to underpinning research in a case study should not be simultaneously submitted in the output component of REF.

(d) The impact claimed has to be linked to a specific output for the underpinning research.

These Are Incorrect

(a) The underpinning outputs can be in many different forms, including non-published items.

(b) The output may have been published after the researcher(s) has left the submitting university, and it could be published under the new address.

(c) The references to underpinning research in a case study may also be included in the output component of REF without disadvantage. The assessment of the impact case study will have no bearing on the assessment of the quality of the output.

(d) The impact claimed does not have to be linked to a specific output for the underpinning research. The expert panel assessors accept that the link between research and impact can be indirect and non-linear.

L. Details of the Impact

This is the most important section in the case study template; it is what will produce the quality

rating; though important, the previous ones are mainly background. Here the impact can be described in an indicative maximum of 750 words, but there is flexibility within the five-page limit. If the word limit is to be exceeded, this is probably the section where that should happen in order to do justice to the impact story.

As mentioned above, compared to the period for the underpinning research, the impact has a narrower time span. It must have occurred between 1 August 2013 and 31 December 2020. When writing the narrative, this time frame has to be borne in mind. There are no marks for 'future' or potential' impacts; avoid sentences that begin with: 'The impact will…', or 'From this we will see benefits in…' or 'It is predicted that practices will benefit…'. Historical impacts that occurred before the start of the census date (1 August 2013) should also be avoided.

In terms of telling a story, this section is where the plot gets interesting. The research impacts can be manifest in a wide variety of ways, take many forms and occur in a wide range of spheres, in any geographic location. The nature and extent of this should be described. What has changed as a result of the underpinning research? There should be an explanation of the process or means through which the research led to, underpinned or made a contribution to the impact. How was it disseminated, how it came to be exploited, taken up or applied and how it came to influence users or beneficiaries?

The details of the beneficiaries should be briefly outlined; who or what public groups, professions, communities, constituencies or organisations were influenced, benefitted or affected? How did this manifest itself and why was it important? In addition, the evidence or indicators of the extent of the impact should be described. These should be appropriate to the case being made and the dates of when the impacts occurred. Where the impact occurred specifically within one country that is part of the UK (e.g. Northern Ireland), this country rather than 'UK' should be specified in the country/countries field.

The REF is an evidence based process and so each impact claimed must be confirmable. Indicators used should be relevant, contextualised and precise in support of the case study, and the evidence should be verifiable and concise. It is important that the impact case study does not under claim, or over claim, what has been achieved. It may be worthwhile to have 'reach' and 'significance' as explicit headings. This will stop the expert panel assessors second guessing the reach and significance. If the impact is a result of public engagement, the narrative must go beyond the reach; the exact significant contribution must be stated and evidenced.

Panels welcome case studies that describe any type(s) of impact, and in most case studies, more than one impact is described. According to Digital Science [8], each REF 2014 case study claimed impact in (on average) three different areas. Questions to ask include: are there multiple impacts and are they all of equal quality? For example, a new pharmaceutical product could have an impact on health, an impact on the economy and an impact of quality of life. As mentioned above, if the impact is being spread like this, make sure that the reach and significance of one or other is not diluted and that the underpinning research applies to all of the impacts claimed. Regardless of the number of impacts, each must adhere to the REF definition: *An effect on change or benefit to the economy, society, culture, public policy or services, health, the environment or quality of life* [2].

Impact case studies tend to be qualitative in nature; they tell a story. However, this narrative can be reinforced with the inclusion of metrics and other quantitative indicators. Making use of such indicators and measures to substantiate the impact claimed is good practise. For example, the qualitative story could detail how a new remote health monitoring technology that emanated from university research has regenerated a poor community and increased employment. This qualitative narrative can be bolstered by quantitative data on the number of new jobs, the annual financial turnover and the number of products produced.

As a means of linking different sections of the case study template, it was suggested in Section I above that references to the underpinning research could be designated R1, R2, R3.

Similarly, as a means of linking the details of the impact to Section M, it is helpful for the expert panel assessors if each impact is designated I1, I2, I3, etc. and the corroborating sources S1, S2, S3, etc. Therefore, when describing an impact and relating it to corroborating sources, the text could include something like (I2, S4).

Here is another task for the reader: the following web link takes you to a 2014 REF impact case study that was rated as being outstanding (4 star). It was submitted by the University of Nottingham and focussed on supporting the regulatory approval of poorly soluble drugs for HIV and hepatitis C. Readers should read the details of the impact section and judge if it adheres to the points outlined above.

https://impact.ref.ac.uk/casestudies/ CaseStudy.aspx?Id=28017

Common Misunderstanding in This Section
(a) That a researcher's esteem is impact.
(b) That dissemination of research is impact.
(c) Some impact types are more valuable than others.

These Are Incorrect
(a) The impact described should not be a praiseworthy statement about a researcher's distinguished career; this is captured in the research environment component of the REF submission.
(b) Impact is not merely about published outputs or presentations at conferences; this might signify reach but not significance.
(c) As with outputs, there is no hierarchy of impact types.

M. Sources to Corroborate the Impact

While impacts described in the previous section can be corroborated from information in this section, these sources should not be a substitute for the evidence provided there. An important fact to remember is that unlike the 2014 REF, corroborating evidence has to be submitted with case studies. In that exercise, the REF team contacted the corroborators directly as a matter of course. While this change has placed an extra burden on universities, it does ensure that the sources are rigorously checked by the submitting unit.

Impact assessors will not routinely be presented with this information. Rather, it will be held by the REF team on a secure submission system and made available to expert panel assessors on request. The information will be used for audit purposes only. So, if the case made and the evidence provided in the previous section are not convincing, the assessors can instigate an audit requesting access to some or all the corroborating sources. The REF team will also regularly audit a proportion of case studies and, as part of that process, it will examine corroborative sources.

Each impact case study can have up to ten independent corroborating sources to confirm the authenticity and the reach and significance of the impact. Ten is thought to be sufficient but it is recognised that in some instances further sources may be required. Corroborating sources can be individuals or groups in the health service, industry or policy makers. It can also take the form of reports, reviews and references to awards and prizes for the impact. While universities may group multiple items of evidence into a single source to corroborate the impact, they must clearly identify and describe each item in the grouped source.

It is also common to see the contact details of individual users/beneficiaries who could be contacted by the REF team to corroborate claims; such sources are not anonymised. For some sources, this may raise concerns about privacy and security. In such instances, their details will be shared via a secure system with panel chairs, members, assessors, panel secretariat and observers, who are all bound by confidentiality arrangements. Because of Covid-19, the revised date for providing corroborating evidence for impact case studies and redacted impact is 1 June 2021. See F above regarding an optional verifiable statement

(max 100 words) that may be provided to explain the Covid-19 disruption on the collection of key corroboration sources.

As stated above, the corroborating sources are often individuals who could be contacted to provide factual statements relating to the impact claimed. In this section of the case study, only the organisation (and, if appropriate, the position) of the individuals concerned and what claim(s) they can corroborate are included. Their personal details (name, position, contact details) must be entered separately on the REF submission system. Details of a maximum of five individuals may be entered for each case study. These are inserted through the submission system data and will not be published. It is not envisaged that more than five individuals will be contacted for any particular case study. The corroborating sources listed should focus on the key claims made within the case study. Extracts from corroborating statements may be included within other sections of the case studies, where appropriate.

Researchers' personal contacts in clinical settings and industry are key to knowing from where the corroborative information can be sourced. Those drafting the impact case studies in the submitting UoA should ensure that the corroborating sources are available if contacted. This can be problematic if there is a reliance on researchers who have left the institution to obtain the corroborating information. It is also possible that individuals in the corroborating organisations have moved on and contacting them can be labour intensive. Corroboration becomes less reliable as time passes and the lack of corporate memory is a problem. Key people in busy external organisations should be given sufficient time and notice when requesting corroborative evidence. Time is also a major factor, especially if the impact has to be ratified by regulatory or legal bodies (e.g. new drug or technology approval and usage).

Submitting universities need to be clear on what exactly the corroborating source will provide to the REF. This should be checked and not left to a hard-pressed external partner who probably will not understand the rules and intricacies of the assessment exercise. It is a good practice for universities to ensure that from an early stage, such end users are educated in what REF impact is, why their help is required and what that help entails. In addition, some industrial partners may be reluctant to corroborate the impact if it means sharing commercially sensitive information or protecting valuable intellectual property.

It is also difficult to quantify the impact of research when technologies have been sold on to third parties or where a university spin out has been 'bought over' by a large conglomerate. What is in it for these busy healthcare executives, entrepreneurs or industrialists? Why should they provide corroborative evidence to help researchers that they do not know or with whom they have never worked? Financial impact can be substantial in the pharmaceutical and medical equipment industries, and such information is commercially (and politically) very sensitive. In such instances, why would the owner of a new pharmaceutical product or a new technology be willing to share commercial information to quantify the financial impact? Moreover, once research is used for profit-making purposes, the company may have good reason to hide its relationship to commercial impact or may be reluctant to supply metrics.

In this section, web links to corroborating information should be used with caution, if at all. As outlined above there are several reasons for this, but they bear repeating. First, assessors will not routinely follow URLs to access additional evidence or information to supplement the submission. The rule of thumb is that the impact case study should stand on its own, and assessors should not have to follow internet links to grasp the reach and significance claimed. Second, web links go out of date or can get corrupted, and if this happens then accessibility is compromised. Third, on average the REF impact assessors may have to read hundreds of research outputs and up to 50 impact case studies. Imagine their frustration if they click on a web link that takes them to a 250-page PDF document, with no indication as to what part of it contains the nugget of corroborative evidence.

Corroborating evidence comes in many forms. It varies across assessment panels and included publications, testimonials, reports, videos, patents and web links. According to Loach et al. [9], testimonials are the most frequently used form of evidence in Main Panels B, C and D, whereas reports are the most prevalent in Main Panel A. They found that the corroborative sources for health-related impact case studies in Main Panel A can be categorised into five types. Around 30% were in the form of testimonials, much lower that seen by the other three main panels. In contrast, around 40% were in the form of reports, higher than that seen in the other three main panels. Around 20% were in the form of published articles, 5% media, 5% intellectual property and 1% awards achieved.

An important point to remember is that effusive testimonials are not likely to provide what is needed. These tend to extol the expertise of the researcher and have little value as corroborating evidence. In many instances, these often appear to be written by friends of the researchers stressing their brilliance. I have even heard of researchers writing the testimonial themselves and asking an external stakeholder to flow it into headed company paper. If such endorsements are used, they should be objective, evidence based and focus on the impact of the research, not how wonderful the researchers are. Such factual statements from external, non-academic organisations would be acceptable as sources to corroborate claims made in a case study. Getting evidence-based qualitative quotes from those who were impacted on by the research is also a good idea.

Corroborating sources are often presented in the form of government policy. Here too, it is crucial to have clear verifiable evidence of reach and significance. Researchers with expertise and standing may have produced results that were taken up by government officials and fed into a new policy. It may seem straightforward to simply include the policy document as one of the corroborative sources. However, while the ultimate impact may be significant, it is often the case with policy debate and policy change that the underpinning research will not necessarily be recognised, cited or referenced. This is recognised as being particularly problematic within the social sciences where informing policy is a likely impact of research. In this case, the researcher should get a letter from the minister or senior official specifying factually and exactly how the underpinning research influenced the development of the policy.

Here specifically I want to mention corroboration for continued impacts. As seen above, these are impacts that were enhanced in some way since the submission in 2014, but with no further research conducted and/or new impact and beneficiaries. For such case studies, the corroborating sources must be very precise in evidencing how the impact has continued in the interim. If sales or the same beneficiaries have doubled in number since the last REF, they should provide the figures rather than simply say that they have increased. If the workforce of a spin-out company has grown in quantity since the 2014 REF, they should provide workforce expertise and numbers. If a clinical intervention has increased the number of patients discharged early from hospital, the corroborating sources should be specific as to what this has meant in terms of numbers and care effectiveness and efficiency. A corroborative statement indicating an increase in the number of patients being discharged early from hospital is not very meaningful. A statement indicating a 200% increase in the number of patients being discharged early from hospital is more meaningful. A statement indicating a 200% decrease in the number of patients being readmitted to hospital as a result of better research-based discharge plans is very meaningful.

Common Misunderstanding in This Section

(a) The expert panel's assessors have access and read all the corroborative sources.

(b) They will follow the web links to see what sources are corroborating.

(c) For multiple impacts in a single case study, a singular corroborative statement will suffice.

These Are Incorrect

(a) Corroborative sources will only be audited on request by expert panel assessors where they have any concerns.

(b) All the materials required to make a judgement should be included in the case study template (REF 3)—no further reading should be required. URLs should only be included for the purpose of verifying or corroborating claims made in the submission. Panels will not follow URLs to access additional evidence or information to supplement the submission.

(c) A single case study often have two or three different impacts. These could be social, economic and cultural. The corroborating sources should be explicit on which impact claim they are substantiating.

2.3 Summary

This chapter focused on the impact case study as required in REF. Readers were taken through all 14 sections, and common misunderstanding were presented and addressed. A bad outcome for a university would be to obtain an unclassified or poor rating for their impact case study. From the foregoing sections, the reason for this may be obvious; however, the following bullet points brings these reasons together. An impact case study may be unclassified because:

- The case study displayed no actual substantive impact.
- The impact had reach but not significance.
- The impact had significance but not sufficient reach.
- The impact was judged not to be underpinned by research of at least 2 star quality.
- There was no clear link demonstrated between the underpinning research and the impact.
- The impact took place outside of the required timescale.

- The underpinning research took place outside of the required timescale.
- There was insufficient information to inform the assessors of the contribution that the submitting unit had made to the underpinning research.
- Following an audit, corroborative sources did not support the impact claimed or the contribution of the submitting UoA to the impact claimed.

See Appendix B.

References

1. Sinek S. Together is better: a little book of inspiration. New York, NY: Portfolio/Penguin; 2016. ISBN 978-1591847854. OCLC 957455007
2. Research England. The research excellence framework; 2020. https://re.ukri.org/research/research-excellence-framework-ref/.
3. Stern N. Building on success and learning from experience an independent review of the research excellence framework. London: Department of Business, Energy and Industrial Strategy; 2016. https://assets.publishing.service.gov.uk/government/uploads/system/uploads/attachment_data/file/541338/ind-16-9-ref-stern-review.pdf.
4. TEF. The teaching excellence framework. Office for Students; 2020. https://www.officeforstudents.org.uk/advice-and-guidance/teaching/tef-outcomes/#/tefoutcomes/.
5. Adams J, Bornmann L, Haunschild R. Excellence is useful. Research Professional. 18 Apr 19, 08:00; 2019. https://www.researchprofessional.com/0/rr/news/europe/views-of-europe/2019/4/Excellence-is-useful.html?utm_medium=email&utm_source=rpMailing&utm_campaign=personalNewsDailyUpdate_2019-04-18#sthash.ceMccvrH.dpuf.
6. Sinclair M. Editorial: what is DORA? Evid Based Midwifery. 2019;17(4):111–2.
7. Rand Europe. Lessons from EU research funding (1998–2013). EU Law and Publications; 2017. doi: 10.2777/667857. Posted on RAND.org on 15 Dec 2017. https://www.rand.org/pubs/external_publications/EP67423.html.
8. Digital Science. The societal and economic impacts of academic research international perspectives on good practice and managing evidence; 2016. https://www.digital-science.com/resources/digital-research-reports/digital-research-report-societal-economic-impacts-academic-research/.
9. Loach T, Adams J, Szomszor, M. Understanding the diversity and value of impact evidence. In: Digital research report: the societal and economic impacts of academic research – international perspectives on good practice and managing evidence; 2016. https://doi.org/10.6084/m9.figshare.3117928.v2.

Research Impact: How to Prepare and Submit Case Studies

3

'What you do has far greater impact than what you say'.
Stephen Covey [1]

3.1   Introduction

In the 2014 REF, the assessment of research impact was introduced for the first time. In fact, it could be argued that this was the first serious attempt internationally. Therefore, to some extent, this was a big experiment and one that was watched by governments in other countries. While pilot exercises were undertaken, the UK was really designing the assessment system as it evolved. The results showed that there were examples of outstanding impact in all universities, and all countries in the world benefited from UK research. This was not too surprising. After all, the UK universities were basing their impact case studies on 20 years of research that had been funded to the tune of many millions of pounds. This is certain but what is less certain is whether expert panel members gave borderline impact case studies the benefit of the doubt. After all, they too were feeling their way.

In the next REF, things will have changed. Thousands of papers and reports have been written about research impact and several in-depth analyses have been carried out on REF 2014 data. The pool of underpinning research may not be as deep or extensive as it was for the first REF. Another question is whether the excellent results for research impact seen in REF 2014 can be repeated or improved open. If the latter is the case, the cost to the UK exche-quer could be excessive. It would be no surprise if the Treasury wanted a wide dispersion of scores for impact. If true, this has obvious implications for how universities prepare for the next iteration. There are other elements at play; in 2014 REF, the submitted case studies often interpreted impact rather cautiously. The guidelines for the next REF stress that impact can be both broad and deep, underpinned by a wide variety of research. It is unknown how this will affect behaviour.

The preparation that universities undertake in identifying and preparing impact case studies for submission to the REF is quite complex. The fact has been grasped that producing the best REF impact case studies requires specialist skills and organisation. There is a growing body of dedicated institutional support, as shown by the seemingly relentless rise of research impact managers, sometimes referred to as research impact officers or champions, a role that did not exist a decade ago. It has been argued that the drive to generate research impact has created an expensive and time-consuming cottage industry within higher education institutions.

Moreover, there is substantial funding directed toward this 'impact industry'. Universities feel obliged to send their staff to the myriad of national research impact conferences and workshops. There are also impact consultants, impact think tanks, public relations firms, dedicated impact

H. P. McKenna, *Research Impact*, https://doi.org/10.1007/978-3-030-57028-6_3

funding schemes, new software programmes (see below), impact leads, specialist impact case study authors, etc. These are relatively recent phenomena, and most have become embedded in university life. Accepting that this is a resource hungry enterprise, it could be argued that universities exist to bring benefit to society, and if the REF did not exist, generating impact would still be core business for them.

The identification of impact case studies begins in earnest at least 2 years before the REF submission deadline. But as research impact becomes more important for governments and funding bodies, this is increasingly becoming an ongoing process. In fact, some impact case studies that are not quite mature enough for submission in the REF will continually be perfected for the following REF.

3.2   Structures and Processes Employed by Universities for Research Impact

One would expect those universities with the best research environment to have the best outputs and impact, but this may not necessarily be true. In the REF 2014, some of the newer non-traditional universities scored better in research impact than the more research-intensive universities. They were very closely engaged with their local communities because they were the institutions that provided the nurses, the physiotherapists, the teachers and the allied health professionals [2]. This may also be due to newer universities undertaking more applied research, whereas the research-intensive universities may undertake more 'blue skies' research, where the impact may be less obvious. Older traditional universities help society by osmosis, with an assumption that their research will have impact at some point in time. Newer universities do not have that luxury because as a young university you often have more pressure to demonstrate your contribution [2].

Regardless of institution type, there are numerous approaches used to generate high-quality research impact; I propose to outline one

that is relatively common. This is best described as being a bottom-up approach supported by top-down leadership and resources. From a governance point of view, there are three levels, with some crossover of membership. These are the UoA level (Level 1), the faculty level (Level 2) and the university level (Level 3).

3.3   Level 1: The Unit of Assessment

The most obvious place to begin the identification of actual and potential impact case studies is at the Units of Assessment (UoA). The Research Directors of these UoAs are, in essence, the custodians of research impact in their department. It is their job to know what research projects are being planned, what projects are ongoing and what projects are complete. From this, they are aware of the planned pathways to impact and the different levels of impact maturity from those completed research studies. This provides them with a good grasp of those research impacts that could be worked up for a forthcoming REF and others that may not be quite ready. Based on this intelligence, the Research Directors identify and support those principal investigators (PI) whose underpinning research would generate the most promising impact case studies.

To illustrate the importance of this process, the input of the PIs is reflected in their workload allocation; teaching and administrative duties are lessened. Just as universities bestow sabbaticals on academics to produce research outputs, it is increasingly the case that sabbaticals are awarded to those PIs who have the potential to produce outstanding impact case studies. The investment is seen as worthwhile considering the potential rewards. This is especially the case in the so-called research-intensive universities.

Yet this is still not the norm across the sector. In some universities, there is a lack of time allocated in workload models for identification, facilitation and development of impact case studies. This failure to recognise and resource the time and effort it takes is short-sighted. For a university to expect its researchers to create and polish high-quality impact case studies alongside their normal teaching, research and administration workload is a recipe for mediocrity. Nonetheless, the allocation of sabbaticals has to be handled sensitively; many academics may think that if given relief from other duties, they too could produce outstanding impact case studies. This often reflects a lack of insight into what is required to generate a 4 star case study.

At their best, the contribution of PIs varies from perfecting existing and continuous impact case studies to considering suggestions for new ones. In this, they are encouraged and supported by their Research Director and dedicated administrative staff. Across the university sector, there are various designations for such staff including: Research Impact Managers, Research Impact Officers or Research Impact Champions. These tend to be senior administrators who have underwent intensive training in the identification and development of research impact. There is normally one per faculty, and they work full time with each UoA, helping researchers and Research Directors to develop those impact cases studies that have the best potential reach and significance. A job description for a Research Impact Manager is provided below.

The number of case studies required in each submission will be determined by the number of active researchers that the university UoA is submitting. These are termed Category A staff members, meaning that they are on the university payroll either as fractional or as full-time equivalent (FTE). For up to 19.99 FTEs, two impact case studies are required; for 20–29.99 FTEs, three case studies are required; for 30–39.99 FTEs, four case studies are required and so on. This formula changes slightly when a university UoA returns more than 110 staff; for 110–159.99, nine impact case studies are required.

However, what happens when a UoA has more than 19.99 FTEs submitted and only two viable impact case studies? Where fewer impact case studies have been submitted than the number required, those that are 'missing' from a submission will be graded as 'unclassified'. The same principle applies at the other thresholds—29.99, 39.99, etc. Such a result would be disastrous for

the submitting university, and it could respond in three different ways. It could accept that an unclassified rating would be given, it could find a less viable impact case study to include in the submission, or it could find a way of submitting less FTEs. This latter option is at odds with REF guidance and is not recommended.

Gameplaying is endemic in research assessment exercise worldwide, but it can backfire on the submitting institution. If it is uncovered through audit that an eligible researcher was not returned in REF, then all the outputs that would have been attributed to that researcher could be graded as unclassified. Submitting universities in this situation may wish to calculate what would be the most damaging to their REF rating—having an unclassified impact case study or having all of a missing researcher's outputs unclassified. The latter would be the better of two unfortunate situations. None of these scenarios should occur because most university UoAs have extra impact case studies that do not get submitted. At the opposite end of the scale, university UoAs should not include more than the required number of case studies.

The Research Directors of the UoAs will know the staffing quota and have a good idea of how many impact case studies will be needed. Invariably (for the reason outlined above), more case studies will be developed than will be needed; these are referred to as surplus or backup case studies. This provides the UoA with a buffer in case some may not be completed on time or others whose initial promise may not be fulfilled. Therefore, some early examples of research impact will flounder and some will flourish. As time progresses, these latter case studies can be honed to perfection. Many that do not make the final REF cut provide good quality fodder for marketing departments, and they often find their way into the local media.

The UoA Research Director chairs regular meetings attended by the relevant PIs and the Research Impact Manager to monitor the progress for each impact case study. The heads of school may also be in attendance, especially if there are workload implications for teaching or administration responsibilities. The number of these meetings increases as the REF deadline approaches. It is at these discussions where researchers hear whether their draft impact case study is to be supported to full development, whether it is to be no longer supported or whether it will be prepared for a future REF exercise.

Once a short list of research impacts have been identified in each UoA, an Impact Writing Team is formed to refine the case studies. This is normally composed of the PI of the underpinning research and the research team members, with input from the research impact manager. As this process develops, a representative from university marketing may be involved. At their best, such writing teams include external research users. In many ways, this illustrates the balance between assessing the work quality of internal researchers and assessing the work quality of external research users. Outstanding impact cannot occur without both investing quality time in this endeavour.

When those case studies that have been targeted for full development are identified, administrators from central university departments get involved. They play an important role in sourcing relevant data sets. This includes the provision of quantitative information that has to be included in the case study narrative. For examples, the university research office provides details of research grants for the underpinning research, human resource department provides staffing contract details, and information technology department delivers research impact software support.

At this stage, a potential difficulty arises. When considering research impact, it is tempting to think of it in the following way. Researchers at University A conduct an investigation and publish the findings, and these make a distinct and material contribution to the economy, society, health, etc. The relevant UoA in University A submits that impact to the REF exercise. This is quite a simplistic perspective.

Reflection Point 3.1 Involvement of Different UoAs and Universities
What complications can arise when the same impact case study is shared by more than one UoA or university?

Different Units of Assessment within the same university can submit the same case study. For example, researchers in engineering, computer science and health sciences could have all been involved in an interdisciplinary project into remote health monitoring of patients' vital signs. They represent three different Units of Assessment (UoA 3, UoA 11, UoA 12). If they could show that **each** produced excellent research that made a distinct and material contribution to the impact, then all three could submit the same impact case study in the REF. As shown in Chap. 2, the UK REF has taken this into account, and each submitting UoA has to ensure that their own distinctive contribution to the impact claimed is specified clearly and that the contributions of the other partner UoAs or institutions to the impact are acknowledged.

The benefits are obvious. Drafts of the impact case study can be shared as can the workload involved. Furthermore, a university would benefit three times from the same impact case study. Consider the importance of this if the impact case study was rated as outstanding (4 star) by the REF expert panels. The funding for this could be substantial for the university. Indeed, it has been reported by Dunleavy [3] that a single case study could be worth as much as £720,000 to a university over the 5-year REF period. Taking the above example, this figure would be tripled. Moreover, it enriches the narrative on interdisciplinary working within that university—an element that will be rewarded elsewhere in the REF. Therefore, it is not surprising that universities are encouraging research collaborations across their schools and faculties.

While the score for the same impact case study is not shared across UoAs, it gets complicated when the impact claimed does not have sufficient reach or significance to support more than one UoA submission. So, if two or three UoAs submit the same impact case study, it could be diluted to such an extent that one or more or all of the case studies could be rated unclassified. In addition, conflicts can arise in a university as to which UoA can submit the impact case study. The Research Impact Manager may need the wisdom of Solomon to settle the matter.

It also follows that different UoAs in different universities could have collaborated on the underpinning research, and hence, they could also return the same impact case study to REF. For example, a pharmacy school and a medical school in separate universities have been collaborating on a research study into personalised medicine. Both these UoAs could return the same impact case study as long as each can demonstrate that their excellent research made a distinct and material contribution to the impact. Here too, each would need to acknowledge the contribution of the other university's UoA.

This gets complicated if the universities are competitive or where it is difficult to tease out the individual institution's contribution to the underpinning research. This is compounded if one university does not recognise the contribution claimed by the other university, or the reach and significance are diluted by too many claimants. As with UoAs, the score for the same impact case study is not shared across universities. However, such salami slicing of research impact could lead to a lower rating by expert panel assessors. The complexity is increased further by the fact that unlike different UoAs within the same university, a cross university impact dispute cannot be solved by a ruling from a single senior faculty or university committee.

A variant on this is also possible: research on information technology in buildings is undertaken by architects in a university and completed there. Health scientists in another university adapts these findings in an investigation into smart buildings for older people. The results of both studies make a distinct and material contribution to health impact. The underpinning research was carried out at both universities, and each can claim a distinct and material contribution to a REF impact case study.

A similar scenario exists when a health science researcher leaves one university and commences work in another university. The research that was started in the first university is completed in the second university. If both parts of the research were undertaken between 1 January 2000 and 31 December 2020, then both universities should be able to claim a distinct and material contribution to the impact case study. The evidence trail has to be presented in each case study, and each university should acknowledge the input of the other. However, caution is urged; if the REF impact assessors are not convinced by the case being made by one of these universities, they could allocate an unclassified grade to that submission.

Once such issues are avoided or resolved, the more advanced impact case studies can be perfected. This may be undertaken by an Impact Reading Team. While each case study is mainly drafted by the academics who were involved in the underpinning research, they may not be able to assess its quality with complete objectivity. Therefore, the Impact Reading Team is composed of academic staff from different UoAs and preferably external stakeholders from the research user community. It is also very helpful to have input from non-experts to address issues of style, presentation and understanding. The obvious benefit of including PIs from different UoAs is that there is shared learning across the university. Suggestions for strengthening the impact case studies are reported back to the Impact Writing Team.

It is also common for the more advanced impact case studies to be sent to external assessors. These are often academics from other (non-competing) universities who have been members of an expert panel in a previous REF exercise, but who are not participating in the next exercise. Obviously, such people are in high demand; they must be signed up for such work early in the process. There is often a fee per case study for this service, and it varies across the sector. For issues of cost, these external consultants should only be asked to review mature case studies.

Reflection Point 3.2 The Role of the Principle Investigator

The preparation of impact case studies at this level requires the commitment from principle investigators (PI). Consider whether this is always forthcoming. What reasons are there for PIs to be reluctant to generate impact from their research. Answers can be found in Chap. 5.

3.4   Level 2: The Faculty Level

As the process of identifying the best impact case studies at UoA level progresses, it is overseen by what some designate a Faculty REF Steering Group (FRSG). This is a middle management committee that meets bi-monthly and is chaired by the Faculty's Associate Dean of Research. The membership includes the Research Directors of each UoA within the faculty and the Faculty's Research Impact Manager. Other members tend to be senior academics who were previously or who currently are REF expert panel members. There are also representatives of the research administrative departments. Occasionally, the FRSG includes some external stakeholders (e.g. health service and industry).

This group is responsible for ensuring that the best possible impact case studies are selected and perfected. To achieve this, there are regular iterations with the Impact Writing Team. Because the FRSG reviews impact case studies across a faculty, they can identify best practice and ensure this is shared across UoAs. This is also the strategic decision-making group. Conflicts regarding which UoA can claim a research impact from a cross faculty project are resolved here.

In the year before the REF submission date, the FRSG is presented with two types of impact case studies; those that are well developed and are a priority for submission and a smaller number of less-developed 'backup' case studies. The former has also been approved by the Impact Reading Team, and central departments have inputted the relevant data sets. The 'backup' case studies will only be used if some unpredicted problem arises with the well-developed cases. Both types of impact case study are assessed by at least two members of the FRSG, and feedback is provided by the research impact manager to the RIs and their teams.

3.5   Level 3: The University Level

Each quarter, the FRSG reports progress to the University Research Committee (URC). In some institutions, these are designated the University Research and Impact Committees. This is nor-mally chaired by the Pro-Vice Chancellor for Research. It is interesting that there is a trend in the UK for these roles to be re-designated Pro-Vice Chancellor Research and Impact. Membership also includes the chairs of each of the FRSG and the Director of Enterprise or equivalent administrator. There are also members representing the central research policy department. It is also good practice at this level to have lay members from the University Senate or Council.

This committee has oversight of the REF preparations across the university, and its members may sample a range of impact case studies to get a feel for quality and readability. This means that they can identify and recommend best practice across the institution. It is at this level that any cross-faculty conflicts are addressed. For example, which faculty should take the lead on or claim a disputed impact case study from a university wide interdisciplinary study. The URC reports upward to the University Senate, which is responsible for research and teaching within the institution.

This three-level approach could be criticised for being too elaborate and expensive in terms of resources and time. However, in UK universities, there has been a surprisingly high level of buy-in among those involved. It is becoming normal for researchers to consider evidence of impact on an ongoing basis and build impact into their research projects as standard. The gathering and review of impact stories is also a valuable exercise in itself. It creates a strong co-ordinated academic/administrative team. It also helps to educate the broader academic and research user community regarding generating benefits from research activities.

As alluded to above, universities are largely reliant on these external organisations and people to create the impact. This three-level approach copper fastens the realisation that research impact cannot occur without the involvement of partners and collaborators external to the university. It is a truism that collaborations work best when all involved gain something from the enterprise. From the university point of view, they have a potential outstanding impact case study that will get rewarded in the REF, and they have met their civic responsibilities.

Similarly, the research end user has benefited from new health interventions, new products, new manufacturing processes or new policies. These are causes for celebrations, and in many universities, there are annual black tie award ceremonies for those who excel at achieving research impact. These are attended by both internal and external partners and other external stakeholders who have the potential to be involved in the development of new case studies.

Nationally, the UK Research Councils also celebrate research impact. For example, the Natural Environment Research Council (NERC) hosts an Impact Awards Ceremony. The awards recognise NERC-funded researchers, showcasing their work's impact in four key areas: economic, social, early career and international. The entrants are whittled down to two finalists per category by a shortlisting panel of experts from academia, business and the non-profit sector.

> **Reflection Point 3.3 The Research Impact Manager's Role**
> It has been stated above that new roles such as Research Impact Managers are now commonplace. Considering what has been outlined in the three levels, what responsibilities and duties would be in the job specification for a Research Impact Manager?

3.6   The Research Impact Manager

A typical job description for such an employee incorporates the following responsibilities and duties.

3.6.1   Key Responsibilities

- Working closely with the academic community and professional service departments to play a leading role in the University's strategy to identify, achieve and communicate its impact, providing leadership on how impact is promoted, measured, captured and curated across the institution and showcased to external audiences.

3.6.2   Key Duties

- Maximise its ability to both achieve impact and communicate it to appropriate audiences, by proactively promoting the impact agenda across the Faculty.
- Work with Units of Assessment and Research Directors to ensure the successful and consistent identification of high-quality impact cases across the Faculty.
- The development of effective and mutually beneficial relationships and collaborations with public, private and third sector funding bodies, research partners, research users, other agencies and stakeholders to maximise understanding and exploitation of University research impact activities.
- Contribute to the programming, delivering and reviewing training and development initiatives of academic researchers and professional services staff (Impact Development Series), through a variety of events, workshops and multimedia on the identification, communication and delivery of impact.
- Work with the University' support services for systems, data capture, procedures and processes in support of the development, identification and recording of research impact activities.
- Conduct analysis of impact performance at Faculty, Unit of Assessment and individual levels, in preparation for the Research Excellence Framework assessment.
- In partnership with colleagues in Marketing and Communication, develop effective communication plans to showcase the Faculty's impact from its research excellence.
- Work with Research Directors and Principal Investigators to identify and enhance impact case studies and report progress at Faculty level.

In many universities, existing administrative staff were redeployed into the new role of Research Impact Manager. Most may have previously worked in the university's innovation or enterprise office. There was perhaps a naïve view that enterprise, innovation and impact were synonymous, and the knowledge and skills required were similar. While linking with external business, understanding spin-out companies, intellectual property, patents and licences are important for some types of research impact, the roles are very different. Researchers from social science, arts and the humanities have little interaction with the enterprise unit in a university. Furthermore, university researchers from the broad range of disciplines may not take advice on how to generate research impact from administrators who lacked understanding and credibility.

The more enlightened university leaders realised this and introduced intensive training for Research Impact Managers. This involved attending relevant conferences and workshops and research impact training sessions. Training includes, *inter alia*, research methodology, the REF process, creating external partnerships for impact, the use of technology and software packages for research impact, and finally, creating, capturing and assessing research impact. These were not knowledge and skills sets that many applicants possessed in their previous roles. In some universities, Research Impact Managers are also mentored by experts from other institutions. These may be individuals who served previously on REF expert panels or whose role was generating research impact in non-university organisations.

While it may not seem central to their role, knowledge of human resources legislation is also important for Research Impact Managers. It has already been mentioned several times in this textbook that as far as research impact is concerned, the stakes are high. To have an outstanding impact case study in the REF is a career boosting accolade for most researchers. It may fall to the 'expert' Research Impact Manager to inform a high-profile professor that their impact case study is not at the right star quality to be submitted in a forthcoming REF. I am aware of one law professor who sued a manager for not including their work in REF 2014. As the stakes get higher and the value of research impact increases with each iteration of

the REF, such a scenario could become commonplace. This could result in challenges, investigations, tribunals and appeals. While Research Impact Managers should be able to offset some of the responsibility to an external impact reviewer, a HR director, or a level 2 or level 3 committee, it can still be a stress provoking time for them, particularly if there are accusations of bias.

Research Impact Managers understand the importance of acquiring evidence of impact beyond academia—on industry, health care or policy. They also grasp the importance of having systems to capture this evidence and link it to research outputs, and of maintaining records of contact with potential users. Some of these systems are described in the next section.

3.7　Commercial Tools for Tracking Research Impact

Not only has the research impact agenda stimulated the growth of new roles and responsibilities in universities, there is also growth in the number and types of commercial tools available. Universities have acknowledged the need for such instruments to archive evidence, plan and provide institutional oversight of research impact. Many have invested in software packages to help them develop the very best impact case studies. The most popular include the Vertigo Ventures-Impact Tracker, Researchfish and the PURE Impact Tracker.

3.7.1　Vertigo Ventures-Impact Tracker

The VV-Impact Tracker Software can store, record and capture research impact and related activities for both funded and non-funded projects. It provides an institutional overview and links to outputs, grants, activities and stakeholders. It is used across many UK, Hong Kong and Australian universities and has been lauded as being very intuitive in the preparation of impact case studies. Most universities that have purchased it have mandated that all potential impact case studies must be recorded using this software.

By all accounts, it is an easy-to-use tool that enables researchers to collate evidence from impact activities and to report the results. It is also perceived as a good learning tool and with its 'Evidence Vault', it fulfils the evidence requirement for the case study. It is a cloud-based software product that has web resources that provide proactive and responsive support. It also helps researchers and impact managers to plan for evidence and report social, economic and environmental impact.

As researchers are working on research studies, they may come across relevant and appropriate online information linked to actual or potential impact. This could include published papers, tweets, reports, videos, images and other media. These can be saved and stored in the Evidence Vault; this is the researchers' personal album for their research project. Furthermore, the VV-Impact Tracker has a 'Web Clipper', which is used to add websites, online images and other sources to the Evidence Vault.

These sources can be linked directly to one or more research projects. It is also possible to ensure security and confidentiality by indicating which audience they wish to share the evidence with or not to share it at all. All current research projects can be viewed on the 'My Projects page', and the content can be edited or removed. Metadata, such as the date and grant reference, can also be viewed on this page. Moreover, each project has a progress bar to display its current status. There is also an advanced option where you can indicate any external collaborators. There are drop-down menus to show researchers how they would quantify the impact and an impact storyboard to store drafts for possible case studies.

It also has uses outside the REF impact cycle as it offers a 'digital shoebox', where evidence can be linked with projects and activities. In addition, it can help in planning pathways to impact for funding applications and in identifying appropriate indicators to measure progress. E-mail threads that are important for a research project,

can be captured and stored and, if required, shared with team members. Researchers also need to schedule calendar appointments and activities as part of separate projects; these can be saved and linked to specific studies in the VV-Impact Tracker.

3.7.2   Researchfish

As stated in Chap. 1, there is a considerable interest in understanding the value or societal 'impact' of research investments, especially those supported by the public purse. While the UK REF 2014 was ongoing, the UK Research Councils and medical research charities implemented an annual impact survey through Researchfish. Formerly MRC e-Val, the approach was licensed to Researchfish Ltd in 2012 to create a federated version of the system to allow it to be used by multiple funders to collect comparable research data. The number of government and charitable research funders that have signed up to Researchfish has increased considerably. It helps them report on research impact beyond academia and inform their future funding strategies.

Researchfish is an intelligent technology to track research and evidence impact. In essence, it is an external system used by the UK government research funding bodies to collect information on the impact activities that are undertaken by its award holders. On an annual basis, researchers and trainees are asked to submit data about the outputs, outcomes and impacts arising from their research. For example, all researchers holding grants from the National Institute of Health Research and UK Research Council funding are required to complete the Researchfish survey.

Researchers have to report any publications, collaborations, further funding, dissemination, impact on policy, research materials, creative outputs, software or technical products, intellectual property, medical products, spin out companies, awards or significant knowledge generated by the research. They are also asked questions on next destinations or secondments for researchers working on the project as well as any skill shortages they encountered when setting up their projects. Researchfish is open to researchers all year round, but there is an annual submission period when investigators are asked to confirm that their information is accurate and up to date.

In 2014, the range of questions in Researchfish expanded to encompass more disciplines, and all UK Research Councils began to use the modified version. It includes data on research awards, publications, collaborations, further funding, dissemination activity, policy influence and artistic and creative outputs. These Researchfish data provide the UK Research Councils with a detailed picture of progress, productivity and quality of their research. Therefore, its role is to convey the quality and impact of the UK research base. The information is worth while in that it is used to inform the UK government's spending review. This is important because when societal impact can be demonstrated from funded research, there is a greater chance of that funding being continued or increased.

3.7.3   PURE Impact Tracker

PURE is another commercial product purchased by many universities across the globe. It acts as a central repository for all academic, researcher and Ph.D. researcher's outputs. It provides live feeds to a researcher's individual and externally accessible 'profile page' consisting of accurate, up-to-date, validated information on all their research outputs, their research grants and awards, their Ph.D. supervision activity and, last but by no means least, their research impact. One of the ways it encourages impact is through making researchers' work more visible and searchable, thus creating opportunities for collaboration and networking locally and internationally.

It is good practice to review and update the impact of your research on a regular basis or as changes happen and progress has been made. Within PURE, there is an Impact Module. As with the VV-Impact Tracker, it can be used to plan for future impact by identifying pathways to impact in a grant proposal. It can also be used to document research impact that is in progress or

has recently occurred, and to update the details, metrics, etc. as the impact matures. A single research study may have multiple types of impacts, and these should all be recorded in the 'Impact' module, accompanied by evidence when available. For this purpose, the impact module can be employed in two main ways:

- To create a single record that describes multiple impacts arising from a project or a series of linked projects, in the form of a regularly updated impact 'diary'. This is probably more beneficial for drafting impact case studies where an impact story is used to describe multiple impacts.
- Where there is more than one kind of impact arising from a research project or projects. Here it can create separate records for each different type of impact.

The impact module is probably best used to establish a single record whose progress can be updated. The Impact Status pull-down menu allows users to record the impact as it moves from planning stage through to maturity. Separate records for different types of impact and/or different impact stages can be created, but users would need to have different titles to avoid confusion and duplicate records. The PURE impact module is easy to use and was obviously informed by the REF. Other research activities can be recorded in the PURE 'Activities' module. These include speaking at conferences, meetings, membership of government bodies or other activities where research findings can be disseminated. Such activities may eventually lead to impact, and at that stage, the two can be linked using the 'Relations' field.

In the PURE Impact Module, the following fields will provide readers with some insight into how it works. As a new impact is recorded, the software asks for the *Title*, which should be concise, meaningful and descriptive of the impact. The next field is a *Description of Impact* which includes who has benefitted from the research, how did they benefit and what has changed or is in the process of changing and can evidence be provided. The next field is *Period*, where details of when the impact occurred is entered. Importantly, this reflects the REF impact census dates. The next field is the *Category of Impact* where drop-down list can be used to categorise the impact as social, economic, cultural etc. The final field is *Impact level*, which refers to the development stage of the impact from engagement, adoption or benefit.

One of the most important aspects of the PURE Impact Module is the section on evidence. A drop-down menu system allows users to indicate if the evidence is qualitative, quantitative or both, a title for the evidence (e.g. company report, publications), a summary of the evidence and a time period for when the evidence occurred. There is also a contact section where the researchers could insert the details of an individual who can be contacted to corroborate the impact during the REF process if applicable or to follow up with at a later point to see if other impacts occurred. The types of evidence can be uploaded to the module, such as screen grabs of websites, company accounts, policy documents, minutes, etc.

There are other less popular impact tools available, but the aforementioned tend to be widespread. However, they are not magical applications; they will not turn a weak impact case study into an outstanding one. In reality, they do not manage or track the progress of impact, that is the researchers' job. Rather they are safe repositories for the capture and storage of relevant data and evidence. There are similarities between the PURE and VV-Impact Tracker systems, but in both cases the information concerning impact will only be as good as the data inputted by the researchers. The disadvantage of Researchfish is that it is tied to national research funding bodies. It will not pick up impact information from studies funded by other organisations or those that have no obvious funder.

But whatever software package is used, it takes time to input the data and academics can get disinterested. However, it can be used by researchers for job applications and promotion opportunities, and they should set aside a period of time each week or month to update the details. It is also useful to build up a portfolio of evidence of impact success for future grant applications or bids. This illustrates how far an academic has come in their research journey and how their research is making a real-world difference. But whatever the preferred system, the underlying objective must be to move from seeing impact as a metric tied to financial gain to seeing it as an essential part of the UK's research culture.

3.8 Incorporating Impact Generation into an Institution's Research Environment

Research impact does not happen by accident. It has been seen above that for outstanding research impact to occur, universities must invest heavily in human, financial and physical resources. However, this is not enough; they must engender a philosophy and a culture of support to enable impact to develop. Part of this is how universities perceived their relationship with wider society. Have they closed campuses behind physical and metaphorical walls or are they open to partnerships and collaborations? Some universities have made this decision decades ago. They refer to themselves as civic universities, or in some cases, they are referred to as red brick universities.

3.8.1 Civic University

One of the first and most famous civic universities is the University of Chicago, but there are many more. In the UK, the Universities of Reading, Ulster and Nottingham are well known civic universities. They have learned how to best manage the array of complex relationships between the university and its many external constituencies. There are a number of ways to achieve this:

- Enrich civil society by harnessing the intellectual capital and the expertise, entrepreneurship, enthusiasm and altruism of staff and students
- Advance an open and fair society through local interventions and partnerships to realise equality of opportunity and access to higher education

- Become an anchor institution regionally to the professions, the economy and the cultural vibrancy of the region
- Be a local to global advocate on societal challenges through disseminating internationally recognised credentials and research contribution for the benefit of civil society

3.8.2 Red Brick Universities

The origins of the term 'red brick university' go back to the Victorian era, when a number of specialist institutions gained independence and became fully fledged universities. While these UK universities got their 'red brick' label from the style of brickwork common at the time, it was their links to industry that made them unique. They include in alphabetical order: The Universities of Birmingham, Bristol, Leeds, Liverpool, Manchester and Sheffield.

Readers will note that these nineteenth-century universities are based in cities that were big industrial powerhouses following the Industrial Revolution. They had strong links with local cotton, linen, and steel industries in their locality, and this influenced the curricula they offered and the research they conducted. Their strength lay in providing highly sought-after skills, training and knowledge in fields such as engineering and medicine.

What civic universities and red brick universities have in common is their strong relationship with external stakeholders. This was underpinned by a philosophy of collaboration, and this led to highly permeable boundaries between partners. This has formed a firm foundation for the generation of impact from teaching, research and engagement. It is probably no accident that these universities were rated highly for research impact in the 2014 REF.

3.9 REF: Research Impact and Research Environment

It has been stated in Chap. 1 that the REF has three assessment components: research outputs (60% weighting), research impact (25% weight-

ing) and research environment (15% weighting). Although this book has focused mainly upon research impact, it can be stated with a degree of truth that all three categories are linked to research impact. The outputs report on the underpinning research for impact and, as reported in Chap. 2, many of the publications submitted in the output component were also submitted as references in the research impact component.

In the 2014 REF, the research impact category was in two distinct parts: impact case studies and impact templates. The latter dealt with how the submitting UoA encouraged the generation of research impact. The submitting UoA had to show evidence that it had a robust approach to enabling research impact, and this was reflected in its strategy and plans for the future. The expert panel assessors had to be satisfied that the approach and strategy described were conducive to achieving impact. In the next REF, the impact template has been incorporated into the research environment category. The submissions will be asked to demonstrate 'the unit's strategic approach to impact and how the institution supports researchers in achieving impact' [4].

This mandates higher education institutions to describe their approach to supporting collaboration with organisations beyond the academy as part of the environment template. They have to produce an Institutional Environment Statement (Form REF 5a) and a Unit of Assessment Environment Statement (Form REF 5b). These must describe the submitted university's and unit's research and impact environment, drawing on quantitative indicators as appropriate and related to the period 1 August 2013 to 31 July 2020.

The expert panel assessors will assess the research environment of the submitted unit in terms of its 'vitality and sustainability', including the approach to enabling impact from its research. The definitions of these include research impact.

- *Vitality*: The extent to which a unit supports a thriving and inclusive research culture for all staff and research students, that is based on a clearly articulated strategy for research **and enabling its impact**, is engaged with the national and international research and user communities and is able to attract excellent postgraduate and postdoctoral researchers.

- *Sustainability*: The extent to which the research environment ensures the future health, diversity, well-being and wider contribution of the unit and the discipline(s), including investment in people and in infrastructure.
- Because it has been recognised that forward planning may be affected by Covid-19, evidence in relation to future impact planning is not expected to be extensive. Assessors will not evaluate the realisation of plans after the 31st July 2020.

3.9.1   Institution Environment Statement (REF 5a)

In this form, there should be detailed information on the institution's strategy and resources to support research and enable impact, relating to the period 1 August 2013 to 31 July 2020. One completed REF 5a will be required for each submitting institution, consisting of four sections:

(a) Context and mission: An overview of the size, structure and mission of the institution
(b) Strategy: The institution's strategy for research and enabling impact (including integrity, open research and structures to support interdisciplinary research)
(c) People: The institution's staffing strategy, support and training of research students and building on the information provided in codes of practice, evidence about how equality and diversity in research careers are supported and promoted across the institution
(d) Income, infrastructure and facilities: The institutional-level resources and facilities available to support research, including mechanisms for supporting the reproducibility of research as appropriate to the research focus of the HEI and to facilitate its impact

In drafting the Institutional Statement, universities can draw on supporting quantitative indicators where these are applicable. URLs can only be used in REF 5a for the purpose of verifying or corroborating claims made in the statement. As with the corroborating sources for impact case studies (see Chap. 2), expert panel assessors will not follow URLs to access additional evidence or information to supplement the submission.

The expert panel assessors will take into account the information provided in the institutional-level statement when assessing the unit-level template (REF 5b). However, in the next REF, they will not separately score REF 5a. Small and specialist institutions that make a submission in one UoA only will not be required to provide a REF 5a statement. However, such institutions should ensure that sufficient information is provided in the REF 5b template about the institution's context.

3.9.2   UoA Environment Statement (REF 5b)

Here there should be detailed information on the UoAs' environment for research and enabling impact for the period 1 August 2013 to 31 July 2020. One completed REF 5b will be required for each submitting UoA, consisting of four sections:

(a) Unit context, research and impact strategy. This includes evidence of the submitted unit's achievement of strategic aims for research and impact during the assessment period and strategic aims and goals for research and impact; how these relate to the structure of the unit.
(b) People, including—staffing strategy and staff development—research students—equality and diversity.
(c) Income, infrastructure and facilities. This includes information about the submitted unit's income, infrastructure and facilities pertaining to research and research impact.
(d) Collaboration and contribution to the research base, economy and society. This includes information about the submitted unit's research collaborations, networks and partnerships, including relationships with key research users, beneficiaries or audiences; and the wider activities and contribu-

tions to the research base, economy and society

The information in REF 5b should only relate to the environment of the submitted UoA and should not replicate information about the institutional-level environment from REF 5a. Submitting UoAs should draw on supporting quantitative indicators where applicable.

As alluded to above, the expert panel assessors will judge both the 'vitality and sustainability' of the submitted unit, including its approach to enabling impact from its research, and its contribution to the 'vitality and sustainability' of the wider research base. Table 3.1 illustrates the five quality ratings that expert panel assessors can allocate to UoAs research environment template. As with Table 1.1 in Chap. 1, outstanding or world leading descriptors are not synonymous with geography.

Expert panel assessors will expect to see how the UoA has sought to enable and/or facilitate the achievement of impact arising from their research and how they are shaping and adapting their plans to ensure that they continue to support the vitality and sustainability of the unit's impact. The submitting unit should detail how the unit recognises and rewards staff for carrying out research and for achieving impact and how the unit specifically supports and enables staff to achieve impact from their research.

Assessors will wish to convince themselves that the research environment of the UoA contains significant features of work conducive to very considerable impact, with some elements of outstanding impact. They may check to see if there are natural partnerships with a wide range of cultural, media and community links both in the national and international context. They may gauge if there is a strong outward looking agenda and effective institutional backing, with clearly identified partnerships and recognition of user groups for the generation of high quality research impact.

Reflection Point 3.4 Staff Development for the Creation of Research iImpact
Every UoA has a staffing strategy and part of that is how they develop their academic staff. What question would you ask to ensure that this was helping to create research impact?

The UoA staffing strategy and staff development policy should indicate how within the submitted unit, they relate to the unit's research and impact strategy. How too does the unit's research infrastructure encourage the generation of research impact? Is there expensive kit available that external organisations use for joint projects? Has the presence of such equipment led to the co-location of new businesses or industries? Has such resources attracted foreign and direct investment? Are there labs and facilities where there has been significant investment for the pursuit of research impact? Have new research clusters been established that focus on distinctive areas of work, which may include the delivery of highly impactful research?

Table 3.1 Quality descriptors for assessing a UoA research environment

Quality rating	Quality description
4 star	An environment that is conducive to producing research of world leading quality and enabling outstanding impact, in terms of its vitality and sustainability
3 star	An environment that is conducive to producing research of internationally excellent quality and enabling very considerable impact, in terms of its vitality and sustainability
2 star	An environment that is conducive to producing research of internationally recognised quality and enabling considerable impact, in terms of its vitality and sustainability
1 star	An environment that is conducive to producing research of nationally recognised quality and enabling recognised but modest impact, in terms of its vitality and sustainability
Unclassified	An environment that is not conducive to producing research of nationally recognised quality or enabling impact of reach and significance

Where is the evidence of how the environment has encouraged staff interaction with, engaged with or developed relationships with external stakeholders. This includes research users, beneficiaries or audiences to develop impact from the research carried out in the UoA and how these collaborations have enriched the research environment. Here too, the environment statement should outline any wider contributions to the economy and society, including evidence of impact from research carried out in the unit that is not captured in the impact case studies.

Many universities have staff who are working in partnership posts with the health service and industry. These roles are referred to as clinical academic careers or joint appointment positions. There are various employment models but the most common one is where a staff member works 50% of their time in the university and 50% in an external organisation. This helps in the selection and development of impact case studies. It also builds trust between the partners so that external collaborators are more amenable to helping draft impact case studies and provide corroborative evidence to confirm the claims made. It also provides each partner with insights into the others' different priorities. While such partnership posts assist in attracting research grant income, ongoing engagement and continuity of relationships beyond the time-frames of the grants lead to continued joint ownership of impact.

Acccepting the negative effects of Covid-19 on future planning, where reasonable, the environment statement may present. Plans on how to continue building and rolling out on the pathways to impact. Is there evidence of growth plans in the impact culture or infrastructure? Are there plans for the enhancement of embedding impact and behaviour change on valuing research impact? Are there high-quality training programmes available on research impact in the institution and funding for training elsewhere? Does the UoA make good use of blogs, institutional repositories, social media to disseminate its research to actual and potential impact collaborators?

According to Research England [4], the submitting UoA should describe how the selected case studies relate to their approach to achieving impact, including:

- The policy for research, impact leave/sabbatical leave for all staff at all stages of their careers (including fixed-term and part-time staff)
- Evidence of procedures to stimulate and facilitate exchanges between academia and business, industry or public or third sector bodies, for the purposes of impact generation
- How the unit recognises and rewards staff for carrying out research and for achieving impact and how the unit specifically supports and enables staff to achieve impact from their research
- Organisational infrastructure supporting research and impact, for example, evidence of areas where there has been significant investment or through the development of research clusters that focus on distinctive areas of work, which may include the delivery of highly impactful research
- Operational and scholarly infrastructure supporting research and impact within the submitting unit, including technical and support staff, estate and facilities, advanced equipment, IT resources or significant archives and collections
- How infrastructure, facilities and expertise are utilised in relation to impact activities

3.10 Summary

This chapter concentrated on what universities have to do to exploit the growing research impact agenda. One lesson that readers should take away is that this is a long and complicated endeavour and has the potential to grow as large as that required for teaching and research alone. Three levels of support and approval were described showing the bottom up approach to impact generation. Each has a unique role in ensuring that the very best research impact case studies are submitted to the REF. This chapter also described the role of the Research Impact Manager and how they are crucial in the administration and governance processes. Three of the most popular software packages to manage research impact were described. While they are useful for capturing and storing research impact information, they will not generate or create impact. Finally, the link between research impact and the research environment was explored. A series of tips and questions were presented on how to show where universities can create and sustain an environment to enable research impact for the REF submission.

From this chapter, it can be seen that there are a number of things that universities should do to prepare for future assessments of research impact. These include knowing the definition of impact and the types of evidence required to show it; educate end users such as clinicians, companies and health services on impact, why we need their involvement, what that involvement entails; involve patients, carers and health service managers in research teams so that they can advise from the start on how the study can achieve impact; develop mechanisms for supporting research impact at institutional/unit level and identify impact case studies early and have them critically assessed against criteria by research users and lay readers. Also, it is a good idea to collect evidence for impact on an ongoing basis. Doing this retrospectively is difficult and time consuming. This chapter told the research impact assessment story from the UoA and the universities' perspective. The next chapter does so from the expert panel assessors' standpoint.

References

1. Covey S. The 7 habits of highly effective network marketing professionals. 2009; ISBN 978-1-933057-78-1.
2. Ross J. Are young universities more focused on civic engagement?. The Times Higher; 2020. https://www.timeshighereducation.com/world-university-rankings/are-young-universities-more-focused-civic-engagement.
3. Dunleavy P. REF advice note 1. Understanding HEFCE's definition of impact. LSE impact of social sciences blog; 2012. http://blogs.lse.ac.uk/impactof-socialsciences/2012/10/22/dunleavy-ref-advice-1/. Accessed 7 Jun 2020.
4. Research England. The research excellence framework; 2020. https://re.ukri.org/research/research-excellence-framework-ref/.

Research Impact: How Assessors Prepare and Assess

4

'The quality of assessors is critical to the quality of the assessment result'
(Pearl Zhu [1])

4.1 Introduction

4.1.1 The Appointments

In the next REF, there will be four main panel chairs and 34 expert panel chairs. These are enlisted through an open recruitment process. As stated in Chap. 1, there are three types of panel members in the REF exercise, full panel assessors, output assessors and impact assessors. These are appointed in phases through a nominations process led by the four UK funding bodies. In 2018 additional main panel members were appointed, including members with expertise in international, interdisciplinary, or the wider use and benefits of research. The aim was to ensure that sufficient expert panel members were selected to make certain that each panel had appropriate expertise for the 'criteria setting phase' (including interdisciplinary research and the wider use of research).

In 2019, UK universities had to complete an Intention to Submit document. This specified as accurately as possible the number and types of staff, outputs and impact case studies they intended to submit. Once this was analysed, the membership of expert panels was reviewed to identify where there were absences of numbers and expertise. When necessary, further appointments were made to ensure the panels had an appropriate breadth of expertise and volume of panel members necessary for 'the assessment phase'. Because of the Covid-19 pandemic, there was a delay in the nominations and the appointment of these new assessors, and the deadline was changed to 7 September 2020.

The analysis of the REF 2014 panel membership highlighted that some limited progress had been made in improving the representativeness of the membership since the 2008 RAE. This included the gender and ethnic mix. In response to these findings and recommendations, the REF team implemented a number of measures to improve the representativeness of the panels for the next REF. These can be found at https://www.ref.ac.uk/about/improving-the-representativeness-of-the-panels/.

As stated in Chap. 1, impact assessors are individuals from outside academia with relevant skills and experience in making use of, applying or benefiting from academic research. They tend to be appointed to the expert panels because of their backgrounds in industry, the health service, the charitable sector, funding bodies or regulatory bodies.

Reflection Point 4.1 Appointment of Impact Assessors
Why might there be difficulties recruiting and retaining impact assessors?

Academic assessors have the support of their university line managers to participate in the REF. In many instances, this is perceived as an important part of their job and to be appointed as a member of a REF expert panel can be a mark of distinction. In contrast, impact assessors are, by definition, busy people in external organisations. They often have significant responsibilities and may have difficulty committing time to the role. This difficulty increased significantly after the Covid-19 pandemic, due to the fact that many businesses, industries and health services were focused on recovery. If face-to-face meetings continue to be discouraged, the *modus operandi* may continue to be tele and videoconferencing. This might also dissuade potential impact assessors from accepting appointments.

4.1.2   The Preparation

Those impact assessors who agree to be members of the REF expert panels are dedicated, and they value the strong relationship they and their organisation have with academic research. Once appointed, they work closely with academic panel members, attending relevant panel meetings and providing detailed feedback on the impact case studies they have assessed and on the REF process.

In the next REF exercise, the structures and processes that universities use to enable research impact forms part of the research environment template (see Chap. 3). There is a requirement that an overall university statement is provided on how research impact is supported and encouraged. This is accompanied by a related statement on how the individual UoA enabled impact generation. This was not the case in the 2014 REF and means that, in partnership with academic assessors, impact assessors may be assigned relevant parts of the research environment template to review. It provides a fuller and more coherent picture when the assessors who reviewed the impact case studies are also involved in reviewing the impact enablement elements of the environment statement. In exceptional circumstances, impact assessors may help assess outputs in areas where they have appropriate expertise.

The impact assessors are appropriately briefed and trained with respect to the details of the REF process and key issues. This includes equality and diversity issues, how to review and score case studies and how to request audits, when required. There is also a calibration exercise before the assessment begins formally. Here a sample of impact case studies are made available and the academic assessors and the impact assessors independently rate each case study. Differences and similarities in scoring are discussed, and when required, expert advice is sought from the REF team. These sample case studies may be from the current REF submission. Alternatively, they may be case studies submitted to another expert panel.

Impact assessors may also join academic assessors in the environment calibration session. In this case, the environment templates may be from a related expert panel. As with the impact calibration, each template will be reviewed independently and any variance in scores discussed. The calibration exercise is a valuable process, and during the 2014 REF calibrations, there were remarkable similarities in ratings across and between assessors.

With their experience of working with research and researchers, impact assessors play a vital role in the REF. Over 250 participated in the expert panels in REF 2014. They were highly respected by the UK's research community, and their contribution was hugely beneficial and invaluable. Feedback from each panel showed that they enjoyed bringing their professional perspectives to the assessment process and appreciated the opportunity to contribute to a crucial part of the UK's research funding landscape.

They also felt that their involvement in the REF provided them with insight into current developments in research that was relevant to their professional lives. It also supplied them with excellent networking opportunities with research leaders and senior professionals in the private, public or charitable sectors. They also gained an enhanced appreciation of the connections that can be made between researchers and external stakeholders and an increased understanding of the potential barriers to engagement with researchers and how to overcome these. In addition, they saw opportunities to encourage a better understanding among academics of organisations' research needs and key contextual information about university research.

4.1.3 The Assessment

The expert panel chair, in consultation with the deputy chair, will allocate work to assessors with appropriate expertise, taking in to account background knowledge and skills and any conflicts of interest. The workload involved in assessing impact case studies will also be taken into account. Each assessor will be allocated a significant volume of material to assess, so that each one makes a significant contribution to the expert panel's overall recommendations.

While in some panels, each impact case study is assessed by all the members, there is a more common approach. Here each impact case study is assessed by at least one academic member (in the REF 2014, this was normally two) and one impact assessor. The academic members assess each impact case study's underpinning research to ensure it is at least 2 star quality (See Chap. 2). They recognise that several groups, institutions or organisations may have made distinct and material research contributions to a given impact. Furthermore, they will expect to see that a submitting university specifies precisely its own research contribution to the impact claimed. When other UoAs or universities have partnered in the creation of the impact, they will expect to see that there is acknowledgement of their contributions.

If they judge that the 2 star quality threshold has not been reached, as evidenced by any of the outputs referenced, the impact case study will not be assessed further, and by default, it will receive an unclassified rating. Alternatively, once the quality threshold of the underpinning research is accepted, this plays no further role in the assessment.

Readers will recall from Chap. 2 that an impact case study can have up to six references and not all of them have to meet the quality threshold. Rather, the assessors must be persuaded that the research as a whole was of the appropriate quality. The research impact component of REF is normally assessed after the research output component. Therefore, by this stage in the REF process, the academic assessors will have reviewed many academic papers. When they come to reviewing impact case studies, they may only read a small number of the underpinning research references to the point where they are satisfied that the quality threshold has been met or exceeded. They may also look for proxies to research quality such as prizes and awards bestowed on the research. In exceptional cases, an expert panel may cross-refer impact case studies to another expert panel for advice. This includes advice related to the quality threshold for the underpinning research.

The assessors evaluate the 'reach and significance' of impacts on the economy, society, culture, public policy or services, health, the environment or quality of life. As highlighted in Chap. 1, the research impact component of REF carries a weighting of 25%. Reach and significance have also been defined in Chap. 1, and assessors will make a judgement about both in the round, rather than assessing each separately. While impacts need to demonstrate both reach and significance, the balance between them may vary at all quality levels. The assessors will use their judgement on this without advantaging or disadvantaging either reach or significance.

As highlighted in Chap. 2, the expert panel assessors in the REF 2014 enjoyed reviewing the impact case studies. These short 4- to 5-page stories of how research had social, economic, health or cultural benefits made a welcome change from the review of books and academic papers. The assessors relished reviewing the broad range of impact types reflecting the strength and diversity of various disciplines. They accepted that there is no hierarchy of impact within REF, and each impact case study was be assessed on its own merits.

Once the academic assessors are satisfied that the quality threshold has been met or exceeded, they will, along with the impact assessor, review the rest of the case study. As with the other components, each assessor reviews and scores the research impact independently between 0 and 4 star (see Chap. 1 for the star ratings). This tends to occur within a set timeframe. Once the expert panel members (i.e. impact assessors and academic assessors) have completed their review, each uploads their scores onto a secure webpage.

The assessors can then discuss the reasons why they provided their particular score. This discussion can take place face to face or through a secure tele/video conferencing link. Following the discussion, they may alter their scores, if required, and explain the reason for doing so. There may of course be differences in scores between the assessors. For example, one assessor could judge the impact case study to be 3 star, whereas another may believe it to be 4 star. Invariably, the discussion will lead to agreement, and the agreed rating will be uploaded onto the web scoring page.

While a rare occurrence, the assessors may not agree on the rating for an impact case study. In this case, the chair of the expert panel will ask another member to review it and provide a rating. This can be an academic assessor or a research impact assessor. The chair may also provide their evaluation of the research impact. It may be the case that the assessors have difficulty accepting the impact as claimed by the submitting UoA. In this case, the chair can request the REF team to undertake an audit of some of the corroborating sources identified in the final section of the impact case study. The outcome of this audit may bring the assessors closer together in terms of their final rating.

While universities can submit case studies describing research impact at various stages of development or maturity, the assessors will only focus their review on the reach and significance of the impact achieved during the assessment period (1 August 2013 to 31 December 2020). They will ignore any impact claimed that is future oriented or that occurred before 1 August 2013. As stated in Chap. 3, such impact case studies are liable to get an unclassified rating. The assessors will also pay specific attention to when and where the research was conducted. As with the impact, the underpinning research must occur with a set

time period (see Chap. 2). In addition, if the academic staff who conducted the research move to another institution, they cannot claim that impact for their current employer.

Because they represent a new element to the next REF, assessors will pay particular attention to continued case studies. These are defined in Chap. 2, and differences in how continued case studies will be assessed across the expert panels can be found in the REF Guidance to Submissions [2]. The expert assessors in Main Panel A will expect to see if and how the impact has changed since its submission in the REF 2014. Obviously, the assessors will have online access to the 2014 impact case study database. Therefore, if the continued nature of the impact is unclear, they may access the case study's previous iteration. In contrast to Main Panel A, the assessors in the other three main panels will judge each case study on merit regardless if it is a continued case study or not. Furthermore, according to the guidance, they will pay no attention to information on how any continued case study relates to that submitted to REF 2014.

Most case studies focus on the introduction of new interventions, policies, products and companies. However, panel assessors recognise that some will lead to a decision **not** to undertake a particular course of action. For example, stopping the prescriptions of a pharmaceutical product that underpinning research has shown to be ineffective or whose side effects are dangerous. Research may also have led to the banning of young people possessing knives, leading to the reduction in crime and murders.

Reflection Point 4.2 Multiple Impacts in One Case Study

We know from the searchable impact database that many case studies describe more than one research impact. Please give examples of where this can happen and any concerns the assessors would have in regard to such cases.

Expert panel assessors will take a specific interest in those impact case studies where several different impacts are claimed. In the REF 2014, numerous impact case studies identified two or three benefits from the underpinning research. For example, a new policy on Covid-19 may have an impact on population health (Health), an impact on people's well-being (Social) and an impact on people returning to work (Economic). Similarly, a new research-based art exhibition may create cultural, economic and social benefits. What will focus the minds of assessors will be whether all these impacts really emanated from the underpinning research and whether the impact has been diluted by being spread across different benefits.

Chapter 6 deals in detail with public engagement, but the views of assessors on impacts stemming from such activity are worth noting here. While universities in the REF 2014 were risk averse when it came to the submission of impact as a result of public engagement, assessors welcome such case studies. However, they will pay specific attention to reach and significance. Almost by definition reach is achievable through many engagement activities—evidenced by audience figures and participant demographics. Assessors will wish to know what the benefit has been or what has changed as a result of the engagement and the significance of that benefit or change.

Another innovation in the next REF is the impact on or through teaching within the submitting university. This was one of the recommendations from the Stern review [3]. Such impacts were not allowed in the REF 2014. Because of their novelty, expert panel assessors will apply reach and significance in the following ways. Here the *reach* of the impact is the extent or diversity of the communities affected by the change in teaching practice. In parallel, the *significance* of the impact is the extent to which teaching practice was enriched, influenced or changed at the organisation(s) involved and/or the extent to which individuals experiencing changed teaching practice were enriched, influenced or changed [2].

In the UK, there is a Teaching Excellence Framework (TEF), which assesses and rewards university teaching and learning quality [4]. The REF assessors may want to assure themselves that universities are not getting rewarded twice for the same quality initiative and that, more importantly, there has been true research impact. Nonetheless, it would be good to see impact case studies submitted that relate to teaching benefits within the submitting university. Assessors may also come across such impacts as part of a wider case study that includes benefits beyond the submitting university.

As stated in the introduction, there are 34 expert panels in the REF, representing distinctive Units of Assessment. Each expert panel is a member of one of four main panels. The main panels are composed *inter alia* of international experts and members of research user organisations. These individuals play a key advisory role in the assessment of research impact. They also participate in a main panel calibration exercise and attend expert panel meetings to offer advice and support. They ensure that there is assessment consistency across the expert panels within the specific main panel and that standards have been uniformly maintained. This represents yet another level of quality assurance and governance for the REF process.

The expert panel assessors also have to determine the overall rating for each submitted UoA. This involves adding the research impact sub-profile for each UoA with its research output sub-profile and research environment sub-profile. The impact sub-profile is formed by calculating the percentage of impact case studies listed in a submission that are assigned to the five quality levels (unclassified to 4 star). Each impact case study contributes an equal proportion to the sub-profile (See Tables 4.2 and 4.3).

4.2   What Makes Expert Panel Assessors Rate Impacts Outstanding or Weak?

In 2015, Paul Ginsberg [5], a physicist based at Cornell University in the USA, carried out a text analysis of impact case studies for the journal *Nature*. His findings showed that terms such as 'million', 'market', 'government' and 'major' were among the words most likely to be associated with those narratives of case studies that were given a high score. Obviously, such correlations do not indicate causation, but they suggest that wording around policy impacts and those associated with economic growth are favoured by expert panel assessors.

Reflection Point 4.3 Reasons for Awarding High or Low Ratings

Please list the possible reasons why expert panel assessors would rate an impact case study as outstanding or weak.

As stated in Chap. 2, all the non-redactable impact case studies from the 2014 REF are available on the Research England website [2]. I undertook an analysis of 310 case studies related to health science (see Chap. 8). From this, it was possible to see why some were rated as outstanding, and others were rated as weak. For the former, the reasons are obvious:

- The case studies told was an articulate, well-written and interesting story.
- The underpinning sciences was strong.
- There was adherence to the word limit and guidelines.
- The statements were evidenced based.
- There was a clear indication of the underpinning research and accompanying evidence for its quality being 2 star or above.
- There was a clear evidence base explanation of how the research results had brought about the change, effect or benefit.
- When corroborating sources were followed up, they confirmed the claims made.

In contrast, a review of weak impact case studies showed:

- Lack of coherence and a dense narrative.
- Journalistic style had unnecessarily 'drummed up' or 'dumbed down' the narrative.

- Focused on the esteem of the researcher and unit rather than the impact.
- Presented dissemination as impact.
- Made unconvincing or overstated claims of the impact's reach and significance.
- The reach was good but the significance was not, or vice versa.
- Intimated that the impact will occur in the future.
- Failed to establish the thread of evidence linking the research to the impact.
- Failed to establish the quality of the research as being 2 star or above.
- Failed to link the impact to the submitting university.
- The impact and/or the underpinning research was outside the set time frames.

These examples, both outstanding and weak, are commonplace across all the submitting UoAs in the 2014 REF. In summary, case studies that made the most convincing claims to impact showed causality, used measures and qualitative and quantitative indicators, addressed issues of attribution and contribution, emphasised progression or spread of impact, showed systematic capture of impact information and presented a tailored account using an active authorship style (see Appendix B).

4.3 Expert Panel Assessors and Impact Confidentiality

All members sign up to confidentiality agreements when becoming members of REF expert panels. This safeguards trust and provides comfort to the REF Team, to the public, the funding bodies and to universities. As has been stated in Chap. 1, the stakes are high in REF; for example, imagine a situation where some impact case studies submitted by a university were rated as unclassified. This may be a common occurrence in the exercise. However, what is uncommon is where a member of an expert panel breeches confidentiality and information on how the decision was reached got back to the submitting university. This might cause them to challenge the process, and it could end up in a tribunal. Regardless of the outcome, such breeches of confidentiality are potentially damaging to the process and its reputation. Thankfully, they have been extremely rare over the 35 years of research assessment in the UK.

While there are almost 7,000 non-redactable impact case studies in the 2014 REF database, there is an unknown number of others that were redacted and have not been made public. Among other things, these may pertain to military research or research that had valuable intellectual property such as new commercial products or processes. These were redactable because once research is used for commercial purposes, the company may have good reason to hide its relationship to commercial impact and may be reluctant to supply metrics as part of the corroborating evidence.

There is good guidance available on the handling of such confidential information [6]. There may be expert panel members or assessors who a submitting university believes would have a conflict of interest in assessing specific case studies. In such instances, a university can identify these when making its REF return, and the case studies will not be made accessible to such individuals. To protect expert panel members from potentially inappropriate exposure to intellectual property, the expert panel chairs may identify specific panel members who should not have access to, or should have access only, to the redacted versions of specific case studies. This encourages more wholehearted co-operation in case study preparation from government agencies and commercially minded industry partners.

For the next REF, due to Covid-19, the revised deadline for the identification of such impact case studies and the related corroborating sources is 1 June 2021. Following the REF, these sensitive impact case studies can be flagged and handled appropriately prior to any public release on the next searchable impact case study database.

4.4   The Views of Assessors and Others on REF Guidance for Impact Case Studies

In 2017, Rand Europe conducted a survey into the perceptions of the REF guidance for impact. It is an independent not-for-profit public policy research institute helping to improve policy and decision-making through research and analysis. Its researchers surveyed those responsible for drafting impact case studies in universities and those impact assessors on the REF expert panels [7].

4.4.1   Views of REF Impact Assessors on the REF Guidance for Impact Case Studies

There was some uncertainty about how assessors would review impact, and this led to unease in the sector. Therefore, Rand Europe sought the views of impact assessors ($n = 555$) on the REF expert panels. The focus of the questions was the level of difficulty they had with the guidance provided on the assessment of impact case studies [7]. Where there was a clear articulation of impact and this was backed up with evidence, the case study was relatively easy to assess. A 4-point scale was used with 1 signifying 'not at all difficult', 2 'a little difficult', 3 'difficult' and 4 'very difficult'.

Approximately 65% of respondents found the contribution of research to impact difficult or very difficult. When asked about judging the quality of underpinning research, 70% found this difficult or very difficult. When asked about judging where the underpinning research was conducted, 75% found that difficult or very difficult. Assessing the 20-year timeframe for underpinning research was perceived as difficult or very difficult for 90% of respondents. For instance, it is possible that the research was 4 star quality two decades ago at the start of the REF census period for underpinning research. However, as science has moved on, assessors who view this through a 2020 lens may perceive it as 2 star or 1 star. Questions about the 5 years impact timeframe also scored 90% in terms of being difficult or very difficult to judge. It is interesting to compare these results with those from university researchers.

4.4.2 Views of University Researchers on the REF Guidance for Impact Case Studies

There was a concern that the rules could be interpreted in different ways, and therefore, universities were uncertain whether they interpreted the guidance in line with the expert panels' analysis. According to this Rand Europe sample, the most difficult part of preparing impact case studies was the gathering of evidence to support impact claims [7]. On a 5-point scale from 'very challenging' to 'somewhat challenging' to 'neither helpful nor challenging' to 'somewhat helpful' to 'very helpful', 60% of respondents found this very challenging to somewhat challenging. For the definition of 'reach', 50% rated this very or somewhat challenging. The definition and concept of significance was easier to grasp but still around 45% found it very or somewhat challenging. The next most challenging aspect was the timeframe for claiming impact. Here 45% rated this very or somewhat challenging.

The concept of institutional ownership of the impact caused some difficulty for researchers, with 40% finding it very or somewhat challenging. Engaging with research users was less problematic with only 35% finding it very or somewhat challenging. Similarly, around 35% of respondents found the clarity around the REF definition of impact very or somewhat challenging. Thirty percent felt that determining the 2 star threshold for underpinning research was very or somewhat challenging. Finally, the 20-year timeframe for the underpinning research was less contentious with only 25% of the university sample finding it very or somewhat challenging.

While these are interesting findings, readers must remember that the 2014 REF was the first time research impact was assessed using the impact case study format. This may account for some of the difficulties and challenges experienced by university staff and impact assessors. Since this was published, a great many papers and blogs have been written about research impact, and there has been a plethora of conferences, workshops and webinars on the subject. Therefore, it is possible that these ratings will not be as high when the next REF is evaluated.

4.5 How Quantitative and Qualitative Data Help Assessors Make Judgements?

The history of science and research tends to be a history of quantification. Galileo famously maintained that we must count what is countable, measure what is measurable and what is not measurable, make measurable. There has also been the adage that if you cannot measure it, you cannot assess it and if you cannot assess it, you cannot score it and if you cannot score it, you cannot fund it. But how do you accurately measure the impact that compassion has on terminally ill patients? How do you quantify empathy, which can have a big impact on a person's well-being? How do you calibrate the impact of person-centred care? So, if researchers adhere to Galileo's teaching, then impact case studies would focus on measuring what is measurable, rather than what counts. What is valued will be securely intertwined with what is quantified and categorised. Such an approach seldom provides the entire impact story for expert panel assessors.

When discussing research impact, Lane and Bertuzzi [8] described the following scenario: *'What worries me is that what you measure is what you get. If you count publications, then you're going to get a million publications. It's like in the Stalinist system—when you had a quota system and you had to produce nails by weight, you got one big nail. If you had a quota system of nails by quantity, you got thousands of tiny little nails. In the capitalist system, if you go to the hardware store, you get a whole wide range of nails. I think we have to respond to the tax-*

payer request that we document the results of science investments, but we have to be able to do it in a way that preserves and fosters the integrity of science. That's what science agencies ought to be focusing on' (page 37).

The very words impact and impact assessment conjures up approaches that involve metrics. Most global research organisations have signed up to the San Francisco Declaration on Research Assessment (DORA), which accepts that bibliometrics are unsuitable for assessing the impact of research on society [9]. But there are other impact metrics. If used inappropriately, such metrics can provide a one-track view of impact, leading to easy-to-measure patents, licences, prototypes, job creation, new kit, number of employees, income generation and cost savings. This is acceptable and works well in some physical sciences disciplines. However when it comes to assessing the quality of research impact, other disciplines are very poorly served by such metrics. These include social science, humanities, art, philosophy, English and some health disciplines like counselling, nursing and midwifery. Quantitative indicators are highly specific to the type of impact concerned. Such an approach runs the risk of reductionism, where a very rich and diverse nuanced understanding of research impact is diminished to a narrow set of quantitative metrics.

UK Innovation and Research [6] recognised that it is not practical to assess the quality of research impact using quantitative indicators alone. They accept that the use of quantitative data to present research impact needs to be seen in context and, more often than not, requires a qualitative narrative and is enhanced by this combination. It is now mostly accepted in several countries that the use of qualitative stories interspersed with some quantitative metrics is acceptable for the assessment of research impact. Therefore, in the 2014 REF, impact case studies were often judged by assessors reading stories, anecdotes, citations and papers, occasionally supplemented by social, economic and healthcare quantitative data.

As alluded to elsewhere, once the REF 2014 was over, a text-mining analysis was carried out on the body of impact case studies [10]. The findings demonstrated that, excluding dates, there were about 70,000 instances of quantitative data mentioned in the impact case studies. Following this, the Higher Education Funding Bodies developed a set of guidelines on the use of quantitative evidence of impact. These not only provide suggested data to help assess specific types of impact, they also include standards for the collection of data.

In summary, where quantitative data are used, for example, audience numbers or book sales, these rarely reflect the degree of impact for assessors, as no context is provided. Even though they are often viewed as powerful and unequivocal forms of evidence, they do not encapsulate the true impact for assessors. Furthermore, they are of little use without their baseline data or control data. Therefore, to be really meaningful for the assessment of the impact claimed, UoAs need to include some qualitative background information. There are attractions to viewing this as synonymous with the mixed method research design. Using qualitative or quantitative approaches alone will only tell part of the story. Using both will bring a richness and an added perspective on research impacts for assessors.

Reflection Point 4.4 Assessing How Universities and UoAs Enable Impact
Readers should also remember that the enablement of research is a core part of the research environment component of the next REF. Here too, the best examples use a mixture of qualitative and qualitative data. Naturally, when presenting such information, one would expect numbers relating to PhD students, their completion rates, the number and type of research buildings and equipment, the quantity of grant awards and their amounts, and the number of professors and contract research staff.

At their best, environment templates will have these quantitative data integrated within qualitative narratives dealing with the research impact strategy.

Qualitative information may include equality and diversity, staff development, collaborations, networks and partnerships with external stakeholders and organisations, human resource procedures for exchanges with business and the health service, rewards and promotions for staff who create impact, relationships with research users and audiences and how facilities are used to enable research impact.

4.5.1 How Quantitative and Qualitative Data Assists the Assessment of Impact?

Research England [2] provides some examples of how qualitative and quantitative indicators can be used to aid the assessment of research impact. I outline a sample of these in Table 4.1. A more comprehensive, though not exhaustive, list can be found in Annex 4 of the REF Criteria and Working Methods on the Research England website.

From Table 4.1, it can be seen that impact case studies employ a range of evidence, com-

Table 4.1 Examples of how quantitative and qualitative indicators can be used to help assessors rate research impact

Areas of impact	Types of impact	Reach and significance indicators
Impacts on practitioners and professional services, where beneficiaries may include organisations or individuals, including service users, involved in the development and/or delivery of professional services and ethics	• Professional standards, guidelines or training have been influenced by research • Professional methods, ideas or ethics have been influenced by research • Professionals and organisations are able to adapt to changing cultural values as a result of research	• Documented change to professional standards or behaviour • Evidence of adoption of best practice • New or modified professional standards and codes of practice • New or modified technical standards or protocols
Impacts on commerce and the economy, where the beneficiaries may include businesses, either new or established, the NHS, private healthcare, agriculture or other types of organisation that undertake activities that may create wealth	• A spin-out or new business has been created, established its viability or generated` revenue or profits • Contributing to innovation and entrepreneurial activity through the design and delivery of new products or services	• Evidence of improved cost-effectiveness • Evidence of service change • Sales of new products/services • Business performance measures (e.g. turnover/profits, trends in performance measures underlying economic performance)
Impacts on health, where the beneficiaries are individuals and groups whose outcomes have been improved, whose quality of life has been enhanced (or potential harm mitigated) or whose rights or interests have been protected or advocated through the application of enhanced health care for individuals or public health activities	• Outcomes for patients or related groups have improved • Patient health outcomes have improved through, for example, the availability of new drug, treatment or therapy, diagnostic or medical technology, changes to patient care practices or changes to clinical or healthcare guidelines • Public health and quality of life has been enhanced • Public awareness of a health risk or benefit has been raised	• Measures of improved clinical outcomes, public behaviour or health services (lives saved, reduced infection rates) • Measures of improved well-being • Measures of improved patient outcomes, public health or health services • Documented changes to guidelines with reference to research evidence • Evidence of enhancement of patient experience
Impacts on creativity, culture and society, here the beneficiaries may include individuals, groups of individuals, organisations or communities whose behaviours, creative practices, rights, duties and other activity have been influenced	• Co-production of new cultural artefacts, including, for example films, novels and TV programmes • Generating new ways of thinking that influence creative practice, its artistic quality or its audience reach • Inspiring, co-creating and supporting new forms of artistic, literary, linguistic, social, economic, religious and other expression	• Testimonials from creative practitioners, curators, media professionals • Publication and sale figures both in the UK and overseas, audience or attendance • Increase in museum and art gallery attendance due to new evidence based policies

posed of qualitative and quantitative data, as appropriate. The assessors will not pre-judge any forms of evidence and welcome submitting universities to use whatever type of evidence they believe is most appropriate to support the impact claimed. This means that a diversity of evidence will be submitted with no one type being perceived by assessors as more important than another. Regardless of source, the role of the evidence is to convince and verify for the assessors the reach and significance of the impact.

It has been mentioned in Chap. 2 that testimonials to corroborate the impact claimed should be used with caution. Those that simply expound the excellence of the researchers rather than evidencing the impact will not impress assessors. Opinion-based testimonials may be acceptable if they relate to public understanding of an issue. However, assessors will look favourably on those that draw on statements of fact and relate specifically to the veracity and significance of the impact. Where a testimony is used as a source of evidence, assessors should be informed if the source is a participant in the process of impact delivery (and the degree to which this is the case) or is a reporter on the process [2].

4.6 Calculating a Quality Profile

Once the three components (Outputs, Impact and Environment) have been scored, the assessors calculate the overall quality rating for each submission, so that it will amount to 100%. The following example describes the process for a hypothetical submission.

Table 4.2 shows that this UoA scored better for research impact than for the output and environment components; 65% of impact quality were in the 3 and 4 star categories. In contrast, 45% of output quality and 50% of environment quality were in the 3 and 4 star categories.

When the weightings (60% outputs, 25% impact and 15% environment) are applied, the situation changes; 27% of outputs are now in the 3 and 4 star categories compared to 16% of impacts and 8% of the environment. Readers will remember that in the UK REF, there is no QR funding for 2 star or below. Therefore, for this example, QR funding will be allocated for 51% of the overall profile (Table 4.3).

The expert panel assessors recommend the quality profiles for all its submissions to the relevant main panel. By doing this, they are confirming that, in their expert judgement, the

Table 4.2 The raw quality scores allocated by the assessors to the three components of the REF

	Star quality (Percentages)				
	4 Star	3 Star	2 Star	1 Star	Unclass
Outputs	17.2	27.6	41.2	14	0
Impact	25	40	30	5	0
Environment	15	35	45	5	0

Table 4.3 The weighted quality scores calculated by the assessors to the three components of the REF contributing to the overall profile.

	Star quality (Percentages)				
Weightings	4 Star	3 Star	2 Star	1 Star	Unclass
60%	10.32	16.56	24.7	8.4	0
25%	6.25	10	7.5	1.25	0
15%	2.25	5.25	6.75	0.75	0
Profile	18.82	31.81	38.9	10.4	0
Overall profile	19	32	39	10	0

overall quality profile is a fair reflection of the research activity in that submission and that their assessment has taken account of all the different components of the submission. Once confirmed and approved, this is the profile that is shared with the vice chancellor of the submitting university. Accompanying this will be a short confidential report pertaining to the submitting UoA, outlining the assessors' views on the strenghts and weaknesses of three components.

4.7   Summary

This chapter examined the review of research impact from the perspective of the expert panel assessors. It followed them through the process from appointment to preparation, to assessment, to scoring impact case studies. Along the way it discussed the matters that they found challenging and those aspects of impact case studies that they paid particular attention to and why. Importantly, it highlighted the reasons why impact assessors may allocate an outstanding or a weak rating to an impact case study. It explored the type of data that they expected to see presented as evidence for impact. The balance between quantitative and qualitative data was described, stressing that either alone may not adequately tell the full impact story. This chapter forms the basis for the next one, which deals with the challenges that research impact brings to both expert panel assessors and university researchers.

References

1. Zhu P. Quality master. 2019. Amazon, Lulu.com ISBN13 9780339254415. https://www.amazon.com/Quality-Master-World-Class-Insight-ebook/dp/B07MWF2B95.
2. Research England. Impact case study database. 2020. https://impact.ref.ac.uk/casestudies/.
3. Stern N. Building on success and learning from experience an independent review of the research excellence framework. London: Department of Business, Energy and Industrial Strategy; 2016. https://assets.publishing.service.gov.uk/government/uploads/system/uploads/attachment_data/file/541338/ind-16-9-ref-stern-review.pdf.
4. TEF. The teaching excellence framework. Office for Students; 2020. https://www.officeforstudents.org.uk/advice-and-guidance/teaching/tef-outcomes/#/tefoutcomes/.
5. Ginsberg P. Text mining reveals REF impact buzzwords Research Fortnight. 12 Feb 2015, 13:56; 2016. https://www.researchprofessional.com/0/rr/news/uk/ref-2014/2015/2/Text-mining-reveals-REF-impact-buzzwords.html#sthash.GlOlbs1W.dpuf Nature report.
6. UKRI. REF: guidance on submissions. UK Research and Innovation; 2020. https://www.ref.ac.uk/publications/guidance-on-submissions-201901/.
7. Guthrie S. Lessons from EU research funding (1998–2013). Rand Europe (2017). EU Law and Publications; 2017. doi:10.2777/667857. Posted on RAND.org on 15 Dec 2017. https://www.rand.org/pubs/external_publications/EP67423.html.
8. Lane, J. Bertuzzi, S. (2011). Measuring the Results of Science Investments. Science. 331(6018):678–80. doi:10.1126/science.1201865.
9. Sinclair M. (2019). Editorial: What is DORA? Evidence Based Midwifery. 17(4):111–12.
10. KCL & Digital Science. The nature, scale and beneficiaries of research impact An initial analysis of Research Excellence Framework (REF) 2014 impact case studies; 2015. https://www.kcl.ac.uk/policy-institute/assets/ref-impact.pdf.

'I wanted to have an impact but also to have a challenge. Everyone can still have an impact in a small scale'. (Souzana Achilleos [1])

5.1   Introduction

Not everyone welcomed the inclusion of research impact in REF. Once plans were released, the University and College Union [2] organised a petition calling on the UK funding councils to withdraw the addition of impact assessment from the REF proposals. This petition was signed by 17,570 academics (52,409 academics were returned to the 2008 Research Assessment Exercise), including Nobel laureates and Fellows of the Royal Society [2]. Therefore, from the outset, there have been critics of the pursuit of research impact, and while many accepted it as an important concept, some were quick to outline its disadvantages.

5.2   The Attribution Time Lag

In Chap. 2, it was stressed that the research-impact linkage need not necessarily be a linear one. In fact, it could be contemporaneous, or the impact can emerge before the research publications are in the public domain. Nonetheless, the REF guidelines allow that the research underpinning impact can be undertaken over a 20-year period (see Chap. 2). This timeframe has generated a backlash from some researchers who are involved in what is variously referred to as 'basic', 'blue skies' or 'curiosity-driven' research, especially laboratory-based investigations. They argued that it is impossible to know and attribute the eventual impact (if any) from their research activities. As Werner von Braun stated, basic research is what I am doing when I don't know what I am doing [3]. In other words, researchers undertaking investigations at the edge of science have little idea of what they will discover. In REF 2014, there was a recognition that this two decade time window may be insufficient in some instances, with architecture, for example, being granted an additional 5-year period.

It was also asserted that the innovations that drive economic growth and wealth creation often depend on breakthroughs in fundamental science. Some of these researchers, such as research physicists and mathematicians, claim that it could take years before their research results show impact. They maintained that such impacts are all but unknown when the research is being planned and conducted. The Wellcome Trust is a prestigious research funding body in the UK. Sir William Castell, Chairman of its Board of Governors, seemed to agree with this assertion. He stated that basic research in the UK is great, but there are problems when it comes to building this huge advantage into a flourishing knowledge economy [4].

For some non-applied research, this is understandable. After all, Einstein's general theory of relativity was formulated in 1916 but required the development of the global positioning system (GPS) in 1973 for its value to be realised. Similarly, lasers were invented in the 1960s, using ideas that Einstein had developed 40 years earlier. Their inventors could not have foreseen that in another 60 years, lasers would have further impact in eye surgery and in DVD technology. This trend applies to other discoveries; for instance, it took around 30 years after the discovery of DNA before technology was developed to enable DNA fingerprinting.

Another example of the research impact time lag was the discovery of penicillin. Applying REF terminology, it has had outstanding reach and significance. It all started in 1928 when Alexander Fleming returned from a holiday to find that some spores of mould from the genus *Penicillium* had formed in an unattended Petri dish. Fleming went back to working on something else, and it took years before others finally converted his finding into a useful antibiotic. It was 1941 before penicillin was trialled on Albert Alexander, a policeman, and it was 1945 before Alexander Fleming shared the Nobel Prize for his discovery [5]. These examples show that time lag is an important issue in the assessment of research impact.

This last example raises another problem associated with time lag, the challenge of attribution of impact. If the time lag between the research and the impact is too long, it may be difficult to link the benefit to a particular researcher or to trace the often convoluted route between research and impact. Even though Fleming serendipitously discovered the penicillin spores in 1928, it was the Australian-born Howard Florey who rediscovered Fleming's paper years later. But it was in 1941 that Ernest Chain, a German émigré in Oxford, tested penicillin on mice. Later, Florey did the first test on the aforementioned Albert Alexander [5]. However, fast forward to the Second Word War when an American scientist Mary Hunt, working in a lab in Peoria Illinois, was able to get enough penicillin from a mould on a cantaloupe. This time lag between the original discovery in

1928 and the manufacture of penicillin in bulk as an effective antibiotic blurred the attribution of the impact. Was it Fleming, Chain, Florey or Hunt? If they were being submitted to REF today, could their research institutions all claim the research impact?

It could be argued that this is an example of slow-burning impact that occurs over time and an arbitrary fixed time lag for assessment may not do it justice. Could it also be an example of continued impact? In other words, Fleming discovering that the penicillin spores killed bacteria in the Petri dish was impact. Chain's use of penicillin to kill pathogens in mice was an example of continued impact. Florey's use of penicillin to save the life of a policeman with a serious infection was a further example of continued impact and so on. Again, in today's REF, all of these could be considered for submission as continued impact case studies.

There are other attribution problems, not necessarily linked to time lag. These include the fact that impact can be so diffuse and complex that it is uncertain what should be attributed to one or other research studies. Impact attribution is further complicated by the international and multicentre nature of modern research. In Chap. 1, it was stated that research impact was a team sport so which researcher, research centre, university or country should a specific impact be attributed to?

An example of where a curiosity-driven researcher may be disadvantaged is Peter Higgs, who discovered the Higgs Boson (see Chap. 8). Such was the precise focus of his research, and the length of time taken to complete it, that for a considerable period he had no published research papers and no discernible impact. Yet when the Higgs Boson was eventually discovered, the impact was world leading. It is impactful because it gives mass to the universe, people, buildings, planets, etc.

This raises several issues relating to the assessment of research quality. First, there is something wrong with a university system that underrates blue skies researchers like Peter Higgs. Second, the time taken to create impact from such research means that some researchers are disadvantaged by a system that reviews research quality over a limited time frame. Third, if Higgs had not discovered the Higgs Boson, he would not have met the publishing and impact targets set by his university, and he may have been perceived as non-productive. So, serendipity has a part to play in the generation of impact.

5.3   Disciplinary Issues and Research Impact

Reflection Point 5.1 Soft Versus Hard Science
There is a traditional view that some types of research are more difficult than others and one discipline's good objective science can resemble another's anecdotal subjectivity. How could such a perception affect the creation of research impact?

In the previous section, the differences between pure research and applied research were explored with regard to attribution and the time lag between the research and the impact. However, there have been other challenges affecting the ability of different research disciplines to create impact. Impact assessments raise concerns over the steer of research towards disciplines and topics in which impact is more easily evidenced. For instance, the impact case studies emanating from social science tend to be on the development of policy. A mix of metrics is required to capture such impact, including statements from politicians and senior civil servants who draft policies. In some quarters, this is referred to as 'soft science'. Because of its narrative nature, the impacts of social science research are often uncertain and disputed.

In contrast, so-called hard science produces patents, new drugs, electric cars, etc. (see Chap. 4). These impact case studies tend to focus on proof of concept, licensing, spinout companies and revenue. Alongside this is the added benefits to business and industry in terms of manufactured products, jobs and share prices. Social scientists and those from arts and humanities may think that generating impact by these hard science researchers is easier. However, they would be wrong. It was seen in Chap. 2 that REF impact case studies use mainly qualitative narratives; a skill that does not come easy to physical scientists. There are other drawbacks faced by physical scientists who wish to produce impactful research.

Some high-quality environmental science studies have to wait for an environmental event before impact can be realised. For example, there are scientists who use complex mathematical modelling to predict the occurrence of tsunamis off the coast of Sumatra. No matter how good the underpinning research is, the impact cannot occur until a natural event happens. If their predictions turn out to be true, the impact is rightly outstanding. If no tsunamis occur, the impact is non-existent.

Taking this example a step further, the impact may well be peripheral to the main objective of the original study. Let us say that the researchers were highly confident that they could predict the tsunamis, and they recommended to the Sumatran government that they relocate thousands of homes from around the coast to the interior. If the government followed this advice, the impact could also be outstanding. But, there is no reason to believe that the Sumatran authorities would take this action. Furthermore, thousands of fishermen and their families could complain that their relocation is a form of ethnic cleansing, a major abuse of civil rights.

Perhaps different impact timelines should be accommodated for different disciplines, with the more applied disciplines having a shorter timeframe than the pure science disciplines. But comparing these disciplines is difficult. One may think that the results of most health research should be able to be directly applied in society. But this is not always the case. When he was the editor of the *British Medical Journal*, Richard Smith stated that the original research into apoptosis was high quality but that it has had 'no measurable impact on health' ([6], p 528). He contrasted this with research into 'the cost effectiveness of different incontinence pads'. He argued that that study was not seen as high value by the scientific community, but it had an immediate and important societal impact. So some health research cannot easily be transferable to patient care due to what Banzi et al. [7] called 'translational blocks', whereas other health research elicits its impact in a more straightforward way.

5.4   A Resource Hungry Process

In his evaluation of the REF, Nicholas Stern stated that the REF should '...*strengthen the focus on research excellence and impact while reducing administrative burden on the sector'*. The REF process has been criticised as being costly: RAND Europe [8] estimated that UK universities (HEIs) spent £55 million to demonstrate impact for the REF 2014. David Price, the vice-provost for research at University College London, estimated that their 300 case studies for REF 2014 took around 15 person-years of work and hired four full-time staff members to help ([9], p. 150). According to the Stern Report [10], the total REF running costs were around £246 million, up from £66 million in 2008.

The counter argument is that this is a good deal; the £246 million represents just 2.5% of the £10 billion allocated to institutions over the REF cycle. This is significantly cheaper than the estimated transaction costs for Research Councils UK funding (approximately 13%). The impact case studies, which accounted for 20% of the overall grade given to each submission, cost £55 million and yet drive the allocation of £1.6 billion over the next 6 years [11].

Universities state that they are challenged by the personal and financial costs of preparing impact case studies. They maintain that there is a significant call on resources to achieve a strong portfolio of impact case studies for submission. These include the time required to draft and do multiple redrafts of the case studies, the time and effort expended in gathering and collating the evidence and preparing the corroborative

sources, the investment in new administrative staff as impact managers and the fees expended in getting mock reviews carried out by external experts. Furthermore, the iterative nature of the impact case study drafting process should not be underestimated. Nonetheless, while the effort is substantial, the specific intended rewards in terms of the QR funding can offset the exertion and expenditure. This is not the case in other countries such as Australia, Sweden and Hong Kong, where the financial rewards for universities from good research assessment are small or negligible.

It is also crucial to manage colleagues' expectations from the outset with regard to the nature and volume of work that will be required. The demands on individual researchers who have to take the lead in identifying, developing and evidencing actual or potential impact case studies should not be taken lightly. It can also be demanding on research administrative colleagues on how best they capture the impact generated by the researchers and continually monitor and refine it; these take time and effort, both of which have a cost.

5.5   The Nature of Knowledge

The Haldane Principle states that the research agenda should be dictated by researchers, not politicians [12]. To do otherwise is to risk narrowing the scope of a nation's research. There is also the accusation that the emphasis on research impact is creating pressures to change the nature of knowledge. In other words, the greater worth placed on research impact, the more that applied research is valued. Remembering that one 4 star impact case study is worth close to six 4 star published papers, the drive for 'blue skies' research may diminish. This trend could steer research away from the imaginative and creative quest for knowledge. This would be a mistake for, as outlined above, in the medium- to long-term, 'basic' or 'curiosity-driven' research may be highly impactful. Furthermore, industries and businesses are more likely to fund research that has easily applied impact and leave it to cash-strapped governments to fund blue skies research. It has been felt that the politically popular competitive start-up culture has undermined the amount of funding and support for blue skies research.

Related to this is the perceived threats to academic freedom and intellectual autonomy. If university management place a higher value on research that easily produces impact, the underlying message to researchers may be to focus on such studies. This could be perceived as a threat to researchers selecting their own research topics and methodologies, a challenge to their academic freedom and intellectual autonomy. Could it cause academics to be more risk averse and less radical so as to avoid getting the reputation of being difficult to collaborate with? Furthermore, could it influence the type of research institutes that get developed in universities and the type of researchers who get recruited, retained and rewarded?

The academic freedom reproach is linked to a prevailing view that universities are turning into businesses. REF and the imperative to generate impact may be seen as just another example of the emergence of managerialism within higher education institutions. It could be perceived as a means of taking control away from academics and placing it in the hands of bureaucrats fixated on income and expenditure spreadsheets, feeding into a prevailing reductionist audit culture.

The focus on research impact could diminish the best of scholarship into evidence soundbites. Therefore, rather than doing their job, academic staff are distracted by countless hours collecting data to prove that they are doing their job. This view is best illustrated by the following quote from Alan Bennett ([13], page 475).

The current orthodoxy assumes that public servants will only do their job as well as they can if they are required to prove it. But proving this takes time, and the time spent preparing annual reports and corporate plans showing one is doing the job is taking out of the time one would otherwise spend doing it thus ensuring that the institution is indeed less efficient than would otherwise be the case. Which is the point the treasury is trying to prove in the first place. Every public institution is involved in this futile merry go round.

5.6   A Distraction from Doing Research

Reflection Point 5.2 Old Dogs and New Tricks

Researchers tend to be highly knowledgeable and skilled, often on a very precise and focused topic. They are expert in their scholarly craft of investigating and disseminating. How does this conflict with and challenge the pursuit of research impact?

It has been stated elsewhere in this text that traditionally researchers did not actively seek pathways to impact for their research findings. This was the responsibility of others, external to the university. This is no longer the case, and there is a growing expectation that researchers will not only disseminate their research but also sell its merits to external stakeholders, managers, practitioners, entrepreneurs and others. This relationship building, collaboration and persuasion take time and effort. For some, advertising their wares is seen as a distraction from actually conducting the research.

Knowledge or technology transfer is often perceived as a staged linear model. The steps are: Basic Science—Dissemination—Design and Engineering—Manufacturing—Marketing—Sales. In this model, the role of academics is traditionally at the beginning of the process. Many are comfortable with this model and confess that they lack knowledge and are unskilled in the latter stages. This is where the hard work of early partnerships with external stakeholders becomes important.

It must be accepted that there are distinct rewards and incentives for the different parties. For academics, they gain recognition, plaudits and promotion by capturing grants from prestigious research funding bodies, publishing in peer-reviewed journals, presenting plenary papers at conferences and supervising Ph.D. students to successful and timely completion. For healthcare professionals, the rewards and incentives are completely different. Their role is to provide safe and high-quality care and treatment for patients and to practise using the best available evidence. For entrepreneurs, the incentives include new designs, new products, capital investment, intellectual property, spinout companies, patents and licences.

The Research Impact movement is disrupting the traditional order of this. It expects researchers to pursue the route to market for their research results and maybe even become a director or CEO of their own start-up company. For health professionals and entrepreneurs, we increasingly want them as members of the research team from the outset, advising the researchers on the best route to impact. Added to this is the possibility that the term 'impact' may have a different meaning for each of these players. Learning these 'new tricks' may be difficult for some. Researchers are almost always driven by personal passion, and getting them to work harder on marketing their work and networking may be seen as downplaying research, the very activity that they are passionate about. Researchers and universities should always remember that the basis of their reputation, prosperity and indeed impact ultimately lies with high-quality academic published work. Getting distracted from this could have serious implications.

5.7   Political Policy and REF

In those countries where there are conservative or right of centre governments, there is a trend towards getting universities to contribute to economic growth and the creation of wealth. Policies are introduced where research for research sake is no longer feasible, and the aim should be to have social impact generally and economic impact specifically. Research review exercises in those countries reflect this viewpoint. In Chap. 9, several examples of this are explored; in the USA, where Trump wants to make America great again. In Sweden, where the focus on assessing research impact was driven by a conservative government, and this was stopped once a new socialist party became elected.

In the UK too, the REF impact agenda has mainly been driven by the Conservative government. The more socialist oriented Labour Party lost the general election to the Conservative Party in 2010. It was around that point in time that the plans for REF 2014 began to focus on research impact. The forthcoming REF, with its higher rating on research impact, has also been planned and developed under a Conservative government.

In April 2020, Chi Onwurah, the shadow science minister and the Labour MP for Newcastle upon Tyne Central, criticised the Research Excellence Framework. She stated that it encouraged a cutthroat environment, feeding into league tables and creating incentives to game the system. She wanted to see universities and scientific research enabling new industries, particularly in manufacturing, that can respond to public health crises as well as decarbonise the economy [14].

Therefore, she did hint at the importance of research impact but did not call it by name. She maintained that academics should be spending their time on research that can inform policy and social change. Furthermore, she wanted to see social and economic benefits from UK research. This shows that even traditional socialist parties recognise the importance of university research having targeted impact, but is not supportive of this being assessed in a REF-type exercise. If elected to some future government, it will be interested to see how they will drive a research impact agenda but not assess it in any regular review process.

5.8   The Difficulty in Capturing Impact Comprehensively

Obviously, the strongest impact case studies are selected for submission to REF. It has always been a trend in the assessment of university research that only the best stories were put forward for evaluation by funding bodies. Therefore, the impact case studies submitted are probably not representative (and need not be) of the actual impact of research in universities. We know that university managers are risk averse when it comes to submitting certain types of research impact. For example, many feel it is too perilous to submit research impact pertaining to public engagement. We know that some managers in university schools of health science have been reluctant to submit impact from some of the 'newer' health disciplines such as occupational therapy, podiatry and nursing. This is based on their belief that these disciplines are on the 'softer' side of impact and preferring instead to submit pharmaceutical, medical and biomedical impact case studies.

Furthermore, if 2014 is representative of the research impact being submitted, then in the next REF, we will see few case studies on teaching and learning, and commercially sensitive and military impacts. So, the impact case studies that are submitted in REF represent a small fraction of the research impact being generated by universities. They will be biased towards impacts that lend themselves to a narrative description and can be convincingly evidenced.

Because of this, early stage impact is seldom submitted for assessment. This does not mean that the research is weak; rather, the findings might be too far from implementation and application. In this case, research impact is just as much a process as an outcome. The ways that science influences society can be subtle, indirect and, as alluded to above, take decades to emerge. Focussing solely on the very best impacts can ignore, devalue and close down other impacts that are perceived as less important or unimportant.

Due to their research expertise, many university researchers are employed as consultants or advisers for policy makers and industry, often informally. In such roles, they spend years providing valuable guidance to businesses, industry or the health service. As will be outlined in Chap. 6, they engender discussions through their presentations and enrich public debate through their media engagements. They also contribute to proper organisational governance by becoming non-executive directors on hospital boards, trustees on charitable bodies and directors of indus-

trial boards. In many of these roles that are having an impact but few, if any, of these activities would be submitted to REF in the form of impact case studies. Of course, this does not mean that REF would not like to see such case studies; it is just that universities are too risk averse to return them in the exercise.

Therefore, we must accept as the norm that only the very best impact case studies will be submitted in research assessment exercises. However, there is a danger that the civic impact referred to above, where most academics are addressing real social need, will become the poor relation to what is perceived as more valued impact.

5.9   Impact and the University Mission

Is the pursuit of research impact really the reason why universities exist or why students go to university? Are not research and teaching the core businesses of universities? What about the importance of universities for character forming and developing individual potential? Colini [15] asserted that 'society does not educate the next generation in order for them to contribute to the economy. It educates them in order that they should extend and deepen their understanding of themselves and the world. They acquire in the course of this form of growing up, the kinds of knowledge and skill which will be useful in their eventual employment, but which will no more be the sum of their education than that employment will be the sum of their lives. It is about extending human understanding, through open ended enquiry' (p.239).

Students in the health professions undertake a particular educational course to give optimum care to patients and further their knowledge and skills. They do not do so to contribute to the social, cultural or economic regeneration of the country. This may occur tangentially as a result of better public health or the recipients of care having shorter lengths of time away from employment. But it is not at the forefront of their thinking or of their career.

Traditionally, early career researchers serve a long apprenticeship where they develop their investigative knowledge and skills. They have time to contemplate their fledgling projects, ask silly questions, make mistakes and learn from them. There is the danger that the unspoken message they are getting from university research managers is that they must pursue research impact. This has the potential to short-circuit the apprenticeship learning tradition of early career researchers.

In Chap. 4, an example was outlined as to how a university prepares for the identification, development and submission of REF impact case studies. This was described as complex and expensive. There is a potential downside to this process in terms of equity. Those universities that are better resourced and more research intensive will invest more in the evolution of impact case studies. In this regard, they may have an unfair advantage over less research active institutions. In such a scenario, it would seem that the REF favours the former institutions. In terms of equity, this means that most of the QR funding goes to the older and more prestigious Russell Group institutions, mainly situated in the south east of England. This could of course backfire on them as they become adept at writing case studies, rather than at actually creating impact.

There is an interesting twist to this story. The results of REF 2014 showed that high-quality impact case studies were submitted by all the UK universities, regardless of whether they were research intensive or not. Chapter 3 described how the newer universities, which were often previous polytechnics, did just as well as some of the older traditional universities. One reason for this is the type of subjects taught in these institutions. The older established ones had a long history of offering chemistry, mathematics, physics, biology, languages, etc. The newer universities offered the more applied subjects such as nursing, media studies and allied health professions. It has been stated previously that the former subjects tend to be linked to basic science research where the pathways to impact are not as obvious as it is for the more applied research.

5.10 New Schools and Departments Being Disadvantaged

For the moment, let us accept that for much research impact, there is a time lag between the study finishing and the impact occurring. This has implications for new university schools and departments. It is an international phenomenon that universities expand and contract as circumstances change. For instance, in the recession of 2008, schools of building, quantity surveying and architecture contracted in size and in some cases closed. In other instances, new schools or departments have opened. In 2019, seven new medical schools were created in the UK. Post Covid-19, there may well be an increase in virology departments or in departments that teach and research on the subject of protective clothing.

Readers should remember that in the REF, research impact is owned by the university and academic staff who move institutions cannot take it with them. Therefore, how could a new pharmacy school or a new medical school have impact case studies submitted in the next REF evidenced by outputs published between 1 January 2000 and 31 December 2020? [See Chap. 2 Sect. C for Covid-19 changes]. This is not possible because the schools did not exist. Some new schools have got around this problem by transferring in some academic staff members who had achieved research impact from their research in other departments such as biomedical science.

Many new university courses have to get approved by professional bodies, and this is a complex and multistage process. In the early years of such new programmes, research quality takes second place to teaching quality and to navigating the journey through the multistage accreditation process. This means that, until they get established, many may not make a REF submission at all. However, this can disadvantage a university greatly in terms of having no QR income for that discipline and the inability to recruit high-quality academics because of the absence of research infrastructure and profile.

5.11 Research Impact: Not Always Good

Reflection Point 5.3 Bad Impact
Come up with three examples of research impact that could be described as dreadful.

Science, technology and scholarship have not always been forces for social benefit. Over the generations, scientists have either purposefully or accidentally created bad research impact. Most wars have involved engineers and scientists developing new weapons. These are too numerous to list here and, in many cases, too harrowing. Furthermore, some wartime scientific discoveries transitioned into peacetime. One well-known example was employment by the US government of German scientists who had developed Hitler's V2 rockets [3]. The results of this did contribute to putting men on the moon.

Nuclear weapons have also been created from scientific endeavours. Although Albert Einstein, a pacifist, did not work directly on the development of nuclear weapons, his research did make such weapons possible. He famously said that 'the release of atomic power has changed everything except our way of thinking ... the solution to this problem lies in the heart of mankind. If only I had known, I should have become a watchmaker' ([16], p 72). But what if a government and a population believed in stockpiling nuclear weapons as deterrents to war. Is a research impact tied to the development of nuclear weapons acceptable and welcome in this case? Should the impact be seen as a benefit or a detriment?

Here is another example, this time related to health care and research on hypertension. In the early eighteenth century, a UK Anglican minister, Reverend Stephen Hales, was keen to research blood pressure. His approach was to tie down a horse and insert a cannula into its carotid artery. The cannula was attached to a 9-ft glass tube. He would then open the artery and measure the height that the blood spurted up the glass tube. While this experiment contributed to a better understanding of blood pressure, a number of horses died in the process [5]. A beneficial scientific impact was achieved for humankind, but in an unethical way. In the history of science, there were many experiments on animals and humans, that would not be approved by research ethical committees today. Do the ends justify the means when science generates impact that leads to societal betterment?

The above scientific contributions were developed on purpose. However, some researchers developed bad impact by accident. The obvious examples here are thalidomide and asbestos. If we take the former, thalidomide was introduced in the 1950s to help with, among other things, morning sickness in the early months of pregnancy. But after bringing about birth defects, it was withdrawn in the early 1960s. Ironically, thalidomide has since been found to have beneficial effects in the treatment of certain types of cancer [5]. But, assessing the clinical impact of thalidomide in the 1950s would result in a totally different result to assessing its impact in the 1960s or today.

For asbestos, it has been used for millennia as a very effective fire resistance material. It found its way into everything from table napkins to the walls of homes. Over the centuries, it probably saved many lives by preventing fires spreading or starting in the first place. However, in our more enlightened times, it has been identified as a major health hazard. Many people who breathed in the dust from asbestos developed lung cancer. To prevent fire on ships, it was widely used as insulation, and many people who worked in shipyards have developed mesothelioma, a deadly form of lung cancer. As a result, asbestos has been banned or strictly regulated around the world. Again, assessing the impact of asbestos before its hazardous nature was identified would differ significantly from an assessment of its impact afterwards.

Another example shows how some impacts can contradict others. In the UK, there has been much research to show that overfishing in the North Sea led to a depletion in fish stocks [17]. The underpinning research recommended a moratorium on certain types of fishing and landing specific types of fish. For fishermen and communities on the northeast coasts of England and Scotland, the economic and social impact from this research was disastrous. For conservationists, the impact was great. How would an impact case study be reflecting this situation fare in REF?

So one person's bad impact can be another's good impact. In science there has been disagreement on this. Thomas Midgley added lead to petrol to prevent 'engine knocking', thus causing health issues and deaths worldwide from lead poisoning. So should the internal combustion engine be improved or should atmospheric pollution be stopped. Which impact takes precedence? Another example from the automotive industry is the fact that batteries for electric cars need cobalt, which is mostly obtained in Sub-Saharan Africa or the ocean floor. Yet another example is where researchers have discovered shale gas in England, a valuable and reportedly inexpensive source of power. But in retrieving the shale gas, minor earthquakes can occur. Therefore, there is uncertainty and disagreement regarding what research impact is preferable (the concepts of agreement and certainty are explored in more detail in Chap. 7).

Many REF impact case studies are centred around job creation. In such examples, new technologies emanating from university research have led to the creation of spin-out companies, and the 'start-ups' have grown over time. This growth has been accompanied by the creation of employment for hundreds of people. No reasonable person could disagree that this is a worthwhile impact. But are these jobs in industries that will damage the atmosphere or lead to climate change? Are they high worth jobs or call centre jobs where low wages are the norm or where some of the materials are manufactured in the backstreets of Bangladesh? So, research impact brings with it value judgements. Most of the research impacts outlined above would score highly using reach and significance as criteria. But what about integrity, equity and justice?

5.12 Conflicting Research Advice and Resultant Impacts

During the Covid-19 pandemic, we saw government ministers on our television screens flanked by scientists. The mantra delivered to the assembled journalists was that the government's policy on Covid-19 is adhering the scientific advice. In the UK, such advice impacted upon the knowledge, beliefs and behaviours of 60 million people. The UK was not unique. Covid-19 was a global phenomenon and so was the assertion from political leaders around the world that they were following the best available scientific research.

The UK government established a confidential scientific advisory committee called SAGE. It was mainly composed of researchers from several UK universities with senior civil servants making up just under half of the membership. In the early weeks of the pandemic, these scientific advisors were strongly recommending to the UK government that 'herd immunity' would be the best strategy. This was based on the view that for some younger people, the symptoms were relatively benign, and they could get a mild response to the virus and become immune. Therefore, herd immunity tended to infer protection on those who did not have co-morbidities or immune systems weakened by old age and disease.

This was not a new approach to dealing with viruses. Rubella, also known as German measles, is caused by the rubella virus. This disease is often mild with half of people not realising that they are infected. However, it can have serious ramifications if a woman contracts it during pregnancy. To build immunity to the rubella virus, often the parents of young girls who got infected would invite their daughters' friends around, so that they too would get this early infection and build up immunity. These were called rubella parties, and they had the effect of providing herd immunity to that virus.

No doubt, university leaders would be delighted if the scientific advice for the Covid-19 pandemic was emanating from their researchers. The reach and significance attributed to such research impact would be outstanding (REF 4 star). In terms of reach, it covered all the UK population and, in terms of significance, it changed knowledge, beliefs and behaviours. While the membership of SAGE was not initially made public, some researchers gained a great deal of public attention for being part of this important advisory body. This brought reflected glory on their research and their universities.

However, it soon became clear that while a policy of herd immunity made sense with a younger population, it had serious negative consequences for the older population and those with co-morbidities. People died in great numbers, especially older people in care homes. As a result, the UK scientific advice changed. The new guidance stressed that the best way to protect the population and curtail the spread of the virus was through 'lockdown' of public buildings, cancellation of events and imposed social isolation. It was clear that in some countries where scientific advice advocated early lockdown, the virus had almost been stopped in its tracks (e.g., New Zealand, South Korea, Hong Kong).

While the 'about turn' and delay in implementing this strategy can be criticised, that was not the fault of the scientists. Nonetheless, they faced condemnations in the media. In essence, the story emerging was that people were dying in their thousands and scientists had got it wrong. Not only was their advice different from the previous guidance, it was the exact opposite. Herd immunity favoured people continuing as normal, whereas lockdown was the antithesis of normal. Could their focus on recommending herd immunity have cost lives, undoubtedly. With the scientific advice stressing 'lockdown', people continued to die in large numbers, and by May 2020, the UK had the highest death rate from the virus in Europe. Contemporaneously, in some other countries, such as Sweden, the government's policy remained herd immunity, and the numbers of deaths there were less than those recorded in the UK.

While the previous paragraphs focused on the UK, the mounting criticism of the scientific advice was an international phenomenon. Both lockdown and herd immunity were based on scientific advice from experts whose research underpinned the outstanding reach and significance of these impacts. The public, business and industries such as air transport wanted certainty. Instead, they got confusion and in many cases, the underpinning research was not made public.

Therefore, at a time when the world needs clear and unequivocal advice from the best researchers, it was not forthcoming. This has obvious questions about research impact:

- Can one research impact that has outstanding reach and significance retain these qualities when it has been replaced by another research impact that equally has outstanding reach and significance? In other words, is one research informed policy less worthy if it is replaced by another research informed policy?
- Could universities claim that they have achieved 4 star research impact, if it is later rejected and is no longer government policy?
- In an era of globally communicated research partnerships, how can one country's scientific advice leading to the creation of outstanding research impact differ so much from another?
- When a retrospective evaluation of the Covid-19 pandemic takes place, will researchers and universities be the scapegoats for political mistakes?
- Has this damaged the reputation of university researchers and the desire to encourage public engagement in science? (I will return to this theme in Chap. 7).

This raises issues regarding timescale. As can be seen in this section, the premature implementation of research-based policies might lead to short-term impact and ignore long-term impact. Furthermore, if impact is short-lived and has come and gone within a REF assessment period, how will it be viewed and considered retrospectively? Is it even possible that a retrospective analysis of an impact case studies from REF 2014 find that its impact was short lived or that it had negative side effects?

On a related issue, is it possible that short-term impact could be the results of smaller investigations and, in some cases, from research that cannot be replicated. Research replication is a major problem in contemporary science and holds particular challenges for research impact. There are many examples of research results that were subsequently rejected or overturned. Could these results be from studies whose findings cannot be replicated, from low-quality research or, perish the thought, fraudulent research?

5.13   Gender Bias and Research Impact

Reflection Point 5.4 The Impact of Being a Female Researcher

Can readers identify five reasons why female researchers are disadvantaged with regard to research impact compared to their male colleagues? Identify three ways to address this anomaly.

In all universities across the world, there exists a gender imbalance, which needs to be addressed. Most senior academic managers and leaders are men; in South Africa, for instance, there are only four female university vice chancellors, whereas in the UK, only one fifth of universities are headed by a female vice chancellor. In Australia, men comprise seven out of every eight university vice chancellors. But what about senior researchers? In Australia, 78% of all professors in STEM subjects (Science, Technology, Engineering and Mathematics) are men. In January 2020, Catalyst [18] reported that the percentage of female senior university professors was 28% in Canada, 23% in Europe and 34% in the USA. There is some indication that this is changing, but the imbalance will not be corrected anytime soon. An obvious question is what effect does this have on female researchers taking the lead on impact case studies.

Throughout this book, it has been stressed that research impact is a partnership between universities and external stakeholders such as industri-

alists, policy makers, healthcare leaders and business leaders. So, what is the percentage of women leaders in these fields? Statistics show that universities are not outliers in this regard. Just 10% of FTSE 100 companies are led by a female CEO, a quarter of the current UK government cabinet members are women, and in one business, national newspapers, a paltry 20% of editors are women. The NHS looks a little better. According to the NHS Employers [19], 77% of the NHS workforce is women, but just 46% of very senior manager roles in the NHS are held by women. These statistics do not auger well for female equity in the pursuit of research impact.

Is this inequity apparent when the 2014 REF results are analysed? Yarrow [20] examined business and management studies, which represented the highest number of impact case studies submitted for any UoAs in the REF 2014. She found that where a case study leader or co-leader was identifiable, only 25% of 395 impact cases were led by women. She concluded that, in this most popular UoA, impact was highly gendered. This under-representation of women researchers taking the lead on the development of impact case studies was also seen in the REF submission to 'historical studies'. More than 70% of principal investigators in those impact case studies were men, and most of these were at professorial level. Yarrow [20] also found that of all REF 2014 impact cases written by professors, 75% were written by men.

It is not within the remit of this textbook to explore the multiple reasons as to why there is a gender imbalance for those REF impact case studies. Yarrow [20] encapsulated the most obvious ones. These include challenges for women with caring and domestic responsibilities, higher teaching workloads and higher pastoral care workloads than their male colleagues. She concluded that because more men in UK business schools are professors, they have more time for research and for research impact.

Yarrow [20] complained that women were being squeezed out of the impact agenda. She called for universities to be more proactive in addressing the barriers blocking women's contribution to research impact. The question is posed as to why universities are not employing impact fellows, allowing women more time to write impact case studies and highlighting the gender balance problem when case studies are submitted to the REF. While these are worthy suggestions, UK Research and Innovation (UKRI), the architect of REF, is very robust in its call for all institutions to respect equality, diversity and inclusion (EDI). Furthermore, as can be seen in Chap. 2, the impact case studies submitted by universities to REF are not linked to individuals; rather they are linked to the discipline-based UoAs.

Therefore, if all universities adhered to UKRI's EDI rules, there would be less gender inequality. As alluded elsewhere, university research managers have a degree of freedom in the deciding on which are the best impact case studies to submit in the REF. In 2014, they also decided which disciplines should be submitted, favouring more of the traditional scientific subjects rather than those new or emerging disciplines that have recently entered the academy. In the next REF, there is a rule that all those with significant responsibility for research have to be included; this should see more outputs from women being returned and them having lead roles in research impacts and research environments.

5.14 Summary

This chapter set out to describe numerous challenges that effect the assessment of research impact. Many of these are due to the fact that such impacts are often unpredictable, diffuse, long term or nebulous and can arise from the messy influence of several research studies by different researchers in different universities in different countries. Add to this the issues around university missions, applied versus blue skies research, gender issues and the complexity increases. Universities have to navigate through these challenges, and if they are successful in doing so, there are financial and reputational rewards. There are other challenges explored in the next chapter concerning public engagement and having impact on policy.

References

1. Achilleos S. Journey to public health science. Cambridge, MA: Harvard University; 2018. https://www.konstantiaachilleos.com/souzana-achilleos-journey-to-public-health-science/.
2. UCU. The research excellence framework. London: Universities and Colleges Union; 2011. https://www.ucu.org.uk/REF.
3. Encyclopaedia Britannica. Wernher von Braun; 2020. https://www.britannica.com/biography/Wernher-von-Braun.
4. Castell W. Welcome Trust; 2009. https://www.youtube.com/watch?v=84cJSPIPa7I.
5. Bryson B. The body. London: Penguin Random House Publishers; 2019.
6. Smith R. Measuring the social impact of research. Br Med J. 2001;323:528.
7. Banzi R, Moja L, Pistotti V, Facchinni A, Liberati A. Conceptual frameworks and empirical approaches used to assess the impact of health research: an overview of reviews. Health Res Policy Syst. 2011;9:26. https://doi.org/10.1186/1478-4505-9-26. PMCID: PMC3141787.
8. RAND Europe. Evaluating the impact component of REF 2014; 2015. https://www.rand.org/randeurope/research/projects/evaluating-impact-component-ref2014.html.
9. van Noorden R. Seven thousand stories capture impact of science. Nature. 2015;518(7538):150–1.
10. Stern N. Building on success and learning from experience an independent review of the research excellence framework. London: Department of Business, Energy and Industrial Strategy; 2016. https://assets.publishing.service.gov.uk/government/uploads/system/uploads/attachment_data/file/541338/ind-16-9-ref-stern-review.pdf.
11. Hinrichs-Krapels S, Grant J. Exploring the effectiveness, efficiency and equity (3e's) of research and research impact assessment. Hum Soc Sci Commun. 2016;2:Article number: 16090.
12. UKRI. Haldane: the principle. Swindon: UK Research and Innovation; 2020. https://www.ukri.org/research/themes-and-programmes/haldane/.
13. Bennett A. Untold stories. London: Faber & Co Ltd; 2005. p. 475.
14. Inge S. Academics should be spending time on research not paperwork. Research Fortnight; 2020, https://www.researchprofessional.com/0/rr/news/uk/politics/2020/4/Academics--should-be-spending-time-on-research--not-paperwork-.html?utm_medium=email&utm_source=rpMailing&utm_campaign=personalNewsDailyUpdate_2020-04-22#sthash.HCb0zAcj.dpuf.
15. Colini S. What are universities for? London: Penguin Books; 2012.
16. Einstein A. Ideas and opinions. New York, NY: Random House; 1954. ISBN 978-0-517-00393-0.

17. Brown P Osborn A. Ban on North sea cod fishing. The Guardian, 25 Jan; 2001. https://www.theguardian.com/environment/2001/jan/25/fish.food.

18. Catalyst. Quick take: women in academia (23 Jan 2020). 2020. https://www.catalyst.org/research/women-in-academia/.

19. NHS Employers. Women in the NHS; 2020. www.nhsemployers.org/.../women-in-the-nhs.

20. Yarrow E. Men define impact as women's research is left out of REF studies; 2019. https://www.researchprofessional.com/0/rr/news/uk/universities/2019/8/Men--define-impact--as-women-s-research-is-left-out-of-REF-studies-.html?utm_medium=email&utm_source=rpMailing&utm_campaign=personalNewsDailyUpdate_2019-08-19#sthash.P1CBazRw.dpuf.

Research Impact: Engaging with the Public and Policymakers

6

'Could anything be better than this; waking up every day knowing that lots of people are smiling because you chose to impact lives, making the world a better place'.

Anyaele Sam Chiyson [1]

6.1 Introduction

The REF has ramped up the requirement to demonstrate the efficacy of our research in 'the real world' where our impact upon the economy, society, health care and culture rather than upon knowledge itself is gaining ground. Everyone from policymakers and health practitioners to the general public is looking for reliable sources of information with which to make decisions. Never before have there been so many opportunities for the research community to push robust findings and evidence to such audiences. Of course, there are many challenges in sharing research through different channels to different audiences. Limited time, resource constraints and the risk of findings being misconstrued or misused are to name but a few. At its best, it calls for academic researchers to communicate in wide range of ways and for the public and policymakers to listen in a wide range of ways.

It is an axiom that researchers present their work to other researchers at conferences, and more often than not, they write academic papers for other academics to read and cite. But in recent decades, there have been calls for academic researchers to leave their 'ivory towers' and engage more meaningfully with the public. Undoubtedly, this is important, but how do researchers connect such engagement with impact? While they have the research findings they want to share, they also need well-honed communication skills and the ability to make complex research results understandable and meaningful to non-experts. But public engagement is not just a one-way communication process. As the Australian Chief Scientist, Alan Finkel, said so elegantly in his address to 'Science Meets Parliament', *'communication is not independent of the audience. Otherwise, it's not communication, it's just content'* [2].

When researchers take part in public engagement activities, they should have impact at the forefront of their minds. The aim should not be to simply communicate research findings to an audience; rather, it should be explicit regarding how, through this engagement, do they change the thoughts, attitudes or behaviours of audience members. Furthermore, they should ask themselves how will they know if they have achieved this aim and be able to evidence it? Without this approach, the opportunities to achieve research impact through public engagement will be lost.

> **Reflection Point 6.1 How Best Use Public Engagement with for the Creation of Impact?**
> What questions should researchers ask before they engage with research end users?

This begins with researchers asking themselves the following questions:

- Who are the people or companies that you need to connect with to create impact?
- Has your university already got links with them?
- Where and when will the event take place?
- When is the best time to present to them and how will you present?
- Why should they be interested in your research findings?
- What are the main messages you want to get across?
- How do you inform them that you are seeking to change their views or behaviours?
- If required, how do you ensure you followed GDPR legislation?
- What support and resources will you need to engage and follow up?
- Once the event is finished, how do you follow up?
- What data do you need to collect to demonstrate impact?
- What methods will you use to collect the evidence of impact?

See Appendix C.

There are some simplistic but effective things that researchers can do to ensure impactful engagement. For instance, if they are speaking at a conference or workshop attended by research users and potential impact partners, they should obtain the names of attendees and their organisations beforehand. A short list of those people with who they must meet and engage should be drawn up. Because much socialising and influencing occurs in the bar or dining room, they should stay in the main conference hotel rather than a more distant less expensive one. They should have high-quality business cards showing their expertise and con-

tact details. Follow-up is crucial, and productive engagement takes time because trust has to be established.

6.2   Engagement and Impact: The Relationship

While some people use the terms engagement and impact interchangeably, engagement is not itself impact. Rather, it is one of a number of mechanisms researchers might employ that could lead to impact. When researchers obtain funding from external organisations such as businesses, industry and the health service, this is at best a measure of engagement, not impact. Similarly, if researchers present to a public audience, conduct consultancy based on their knowledge of the field, participate in a science festival or engage in outreach; this is also more likely to be 'engagement' rather than 'impact. It is interesting that the Australian equivalent of REF recognised this dichotomy and made impact and engagement separate entities within its Excellence in Research for Australia (ERA) system (see Chap. 9). It recognises that engagement is important as an independent activity and one that can hasten the generation of research impact. In the UK, engagement is rewarded through the Knowledge Exchange Framework (KEF) [3] rather than explicitly through REF.

Within the REF exercise, impact from public engagement may represent the main focus in a REF case study or be one part of a wider impact. Regardless, UK universities have been reluctant to submit such impact case studies to REF. This is despite the fact that funding bodies and expert panel assessors want to see impact being created through public engagement. In the 2014 REF, the expert panels did get a small number of public engagement impacts. Such impacts were innovative, valuable and just as capable of being of outstanding quality as any other type of impact submitted.

The reservations that institutions have are linked to concerns about how public engagement impacts might be evidenced by Units of Assessment (UoA) and assessed by expert panel members. After all, impact relating to a new product, an increase in income or a new policy is easier to evidence than how public engagement caused a change in the way people thought, understood or behaved.

As with all REF impact case studies, those that are a result of public engagement must show that the impact was materially and distinctly related to the underpinning research conducted in the submitting university. Furthermore, reach and significance are crucial criteria for public engagement. While the audience participant figures may show that reach was outstanding, what really changed as a result of this public engagement? It could be argued that public engagement without evidence of significance is little more than dissemination. But proving reach might also be a challenge; the audience may be small, unrepresentative or inappropriate. So, researchers have to be creative if they want to evidence their public engagement activities. For example, the number of attendees at an event may provide an indication of the reach of the impact. In this example, significance might be evidenced through participant feedback, post-conference surveys, social media hits, media reports or critical reviews.

It is important to remember that if researchers are collecting personal information to evidence reach and significance, they have to adhere to the General Data Protection Regulation (GDPR). Not only must the data be handled properly and stored securely, they must inform the attendees: what data are being collected, what they will be used for, whether they will be shared with others, where and how they are stored, that storage will be password protected, that their consent is required, that they can opt out at any time and that printouts of attendees will not be used. This can be off putting for some researchers, and they should consider using one of the many experienced event-organising companies such as Getinvited or Eventbrite.

Professor Brian Cox from Manchester University is an expert at bringing complex science to the public. He is a talented communicator who presents a number of popular UK television programmes about physics and space. He reaches millions of viewers through this medium, but

how does he match this reach with significance? One of the methods he uses is to go into schools and discuss the science with children in an interactive and understandable way, using examples that are meaningful to them. As a result, school children participate in science projects and related homework. This provides evidence of significance, as it changes the thinking, knowledge and behaviour of the children, which may also have a ripple effect with their parents.

There is another instance where public engagement can create impact. This is where an academic expert takes on a consultancy role with companies or other types of external organisations. In this example, the researcher is not presenting to an audience or conference delegates; rather, they are providing professional advice or expert testimony. Such advice or testimony could lead to the development of a new product or a new manufacturing process. However, the submitting unit must show that the researcher's appointment to their advisory role, or the specific advice given, was at least in part based on the submitted unit's research and drew materially and distinctly upon it.

As alluded to above, this approach to creating research impact is especially pertinent in the humanities and social sciences where there is a long tradition for intellectuals, scholars and researchers influencing the direction of policy and strategy, which feeds into societal benefit. For example, social scientists whose research is focused on population growth may be asked by a local city council to advise them on the site for a new primary school. Their expertise on the local population, its age groupings, family sizes, mobility and other demographic details influences the council's plans, and the school gets the go ahead for the preferred location. This result shows a direct link to the underpinning research, and the reach and significance can be evidenced.

Expert university advisors and consultants can also influence impact from the physical sciences. Let us suppose that metallurgy scientists from a local university were employed as consultants by a large multinational mining company to provide advice on how best to identify sites where there are gold deposits. The scientists draw substantially on the research conducted within their university's UoA. By using research-based technologies and reagents on soil samples and mineral deposits from a variety of sites, they can assert with a high degree of certainty where drilling should take place. The mining company uses this technology and knowhow in various parts of the world as a reliable and valid method to detect prospective gold deposits. In this example, the expertise gained through university research has had reach and significance. This approach to public engagement is common in universities but, as with public engagement generally, not many examples have been submitted as impact case studies in the REF.

Another example of pubic engagement through external consultancy relates to the response to the Covid-19 pandemic. As advisors to their governments, university researchers provided a great deal of assurance and comfort to the public that the governments' handling of the pandemic was based on the best available research. Each daily press briefing was a public engagement event, and the outcome affected the behaviour of entire populations. The crisis engendered a greed for the latest research on how people should avoid being infected. Seldom before, did researchers take centre stage in terms of global engagement.

6.3   Research Advice on Covid-19 and Its Effect on Public Engagement

In the next chapter, I refer to certainty and agreement; these are criteria the public cry out for from science. However, researchers disagree all the time, and this is an acceptable aspect of academic life. One view on an issue is often rebutted by another equally valid view and researchers challenge other researchers on topics such as their use of sampling, statistics and scales. The public have not always grasped that debate over research results is the norm in science. But, as I outlined in Chap. 5, there were problems with how the public perceived research disagreement with regard to Covid-19.

For public engagement, an opportunity was tarnished by the perceptions that researchers opposed each other as to the best approach to avoid contracting the virus. Furthermore, the best scientific advice in the UK (e.g. Lockdown) was at odds with the best scientific advice in Sweden (e.g. Herd Immunity). Civil servants appeared to influence what science was communicated to ministers. This caused journalists, media commentators and opposition politicians to distrust the advice, and across the world, there were demonstrations calling for the cessation of lockdown. According to a senior Swedish research leader, trust in science eroded as scientists get drawn into messy, polarised debates and rather than exposure to science making politics better, it seems that exposure to politics is making science worse [4].

In an ideal world, the best research advice is required and should not be overturned by new advice; this confuses the public and weakens their confidence in the underpinning research and the researchers. Another lesson is that the expert scientific advice should not be filtered by non-scientific civil servants. As has been outlined above, for public engagement impact, the science is not enough, and communication skills and trust are other important components in the process. This was not helped by the realisation in May 2020 that Professor Neil Ferguson, the Imperial College London epidemiologist, who recommended lockdown in the UK, broke the lockdown rules himself.

Researchers were not to blame; most did not seek to exert such influence and control over the population. Politicians and unelected senior government officials asked them for guidance based on the best evidence. The government decided to follow the advice, and as data increases, it informs the science, and the advice can change. This basic rule of science has not been adequately explained to, or accepted by the public, and the scientists are in the firing line. In Germany, Christian Drosten scientific advisor to German leaders was pilloried in the press because of his advice, as was Anders Tegnellin, the Swedish government advisor. When evaluations of governments' responses to the pandemic are conducted, it is possible that the scientists will be scapegoated and blamed. The effect of this on public engagement with researchers is yet to be established, but it may not be good.

Referring to the Covid-19 pandemic, Aksoy et al. [5] asserted that there is a divide between what scientists recommend and the perception of the public. While scientists have to advise those in charge, if they fail to explain their findings clearly and concisely and fail to inspire trust, the public will probably see them as elitists or inaccessible. They maintain that if politicians use science as a facade of authority and as a scapegoat, the public will eventually blame scientists for not being able to deal with the problem in an effective way. It is less than a decade ago that Italian research seismologists were jailed because they had not predicted the devastating L'Aquila earthquake [6].

6.4   Bodies that Assist Public Engagement

To enhance impact from public engagement, governments need to incentivise researchers with targeted ring-fenced funding. One such scheme does this in the UK. In April 2019 the research councils provided funding to universities for knowledge exchange and engagement activities through Impact Acceleration Accounts (IAAs). These are block awards made to research organisations to accelerate the impact of research. The funding lasts for 4 years. It allows research organisations to respond to impact opportunities in more flexible, responsive and creative ways. It strengthens engagement between researchers and research users, supports new, innovative and imaginative approaches to knowledge exchange and impact and strengthens research organisations' knowledge exchange through raising researchers' awareness, skills and confidence.

Another resource is the National Co-ordinating Centre for Public Engagement [7]. It offers excellent guides on how to organise public engagement activities. These guides cover many areas such as target audiences, methods of engaging members of the public and how to successfully evaluate your projects. The NCCPE identified three broad

pathways to public engagement impact. These are: understanding (exploring meaning and values); capability (enhancing skills, behaviour and networks) and innovation (improving policies and practice and the way the world works).

Reflection Point 6.2 Identification of Networks for Generating Research Impact
In essence, research impact is created through partnership between researcher and end users of the research. Most researchers who are experts in their field know how to connect to external stakeholders. For those that do not, a number of strategies can be used. When I refer to impacts on policymaking below, readers will note that many governments have established fora to encourage links with researchers. Similarly, most universities have research institutes with established networks with policymakers, healthcare providers, industry and business. Researchers should be able to access these networks to enable their research to have impact. They should also make use of their university consultancy office to identify potential end users for their findings. These offices have well-established and trusting connections with the external organisations.

Researchers should not underestimate the value of luck and cold calling. Social media can also play a part, and LinkedIn specialises in bringing interested parties together for mutual benefit. Serendipitous social events can also lead to engagement for impact. However, people can often guard their networks jealously. After all they may have taken years to foster. Academics in particular can be reluctant to share their valuable networks with colleagues. This may be due to a fear that a third party could damage the wonderful working relationship that they have with a research end user. One solution would be to involve these well-connected academic colleagues in the creation of the impact.

6.5   Social Media and Altmetrics as Tools for Impact

Another means of evaluating the impact of public engagement is through altmetrics. This is a term coined in 2010 by ImpactStory co-founder Jason Priem [8]. It refers to a range of measures of research impact that go beyond citations. Altmetrics are based on the number of times an article is shared, downloaded or mentioned on social media, blogs or in newspapers or in scholarly and scientific publishing. They are an alternative to the widely used journal impact factor and personal citation indices such as the h-index. They enable scientists to see ripples generated by their research that might otherwise go unnoticed. Its aim is to track and measure the social impact of scientific publications and the researcher influence [9]. However, it is unclear whether they really capture or reflect societal impact.

People who attend researchers' presentations or read their research articles may blog about it, retweet it and disseminate the findings through other social media outlets. It cannot be denied that this increases public engagement with the research. However, how does the researcher establish that such increased reach has had significance? One way may be to analyse those social media activities that show a change in people's attitudes, thinking and behaviour.

For example, sport and exercise researchers may publish and present their findings on how 10,000 steps each day had a positive effect on people's mental health. This could generate a Twitter storm and numerous Facebook comments on how people had tried this and their mental health had improved. These altmetrics showed both reach (number of people engaging) and significance (the reported positive effect) could form the basis for an impact case study.

However, this is not definitive. Bornmann et al. [10] conducted a study on altmetrics, citation counts, research outputs and case study data from the 2014 UK REF. They also included peers' REF assessments of research outputs and societal impacts. Two sets of data were used: publications submitted in the outputs category to the REF (PRO) and publications referenced in impact case studies (PCS). The findings suggested that altmetrics may capture a different aspect of societal impact, which the authors called 'unknown attention'. This was different from that required by REF impact assessors, who are interested in the causal link between research and societal benefit. Previously, Loach et al. [11] interviewed a range of experts but found no clear link between altmetrics and economic, social or professional impact. They concluded that altmetric scores do not reflect wider economic, social, cultural or policy impact. They suggested that altmetrics should not be used as markers of societal impact.

The same team found that tweets do not appear to reflect any serious form of impact. Furthermore, they compared altmetrics with the scores of REF reviewers for each disciplinary panel and submitting institution. They found that the REF scores of impact case studies correlated only weekly with altmetrics—suggesting, once again, that these measures should not be used as markers of impact [12].

To conclude this section, it can be stated with a degree of certainty that reach is relatively easy to estimate in public engagement activities. Audience participation figures, member lists of public bodies and conference attendance directories are just some of the tools that can be used. However, researchers need to get resourceful in gauging significance from public engagement. Otherwise, universities will continue to be risk averse when it comes to submitting such impact case studies to the REF. It also showed how public engagement for impact can be undermined by conflicting results and lack of trust in science. Finally, altmetrics may be a good mechanism for increasing reach, but there are problems in establishing significance.

6.6   Research Impact and Policymaking

In Chap. 7, the link between evidence-informed practice and research impact is explored. It is concluded that they are not the same thing. The same applied to evidence-informed policy. It is a necessary step towards impact but not sufficient on its own to be impact. Florence Nightingale once said that reports are not self-executive. The same can be said of policies. On their own they are of little benefit, but when they are implemented and positive change occurs, they can be impactful. There is no agreed meaning on what policy is. It has been defined as a course or principle of action adopted or proposed by a government, party, business or individual [13]. This is an important definition as it reminds us that policies are also used in business, healthcare and industrial organisations, and researchers can achieve impact by influencing and changing such policies.

Governments need evidence-informed policy, and researchers have always been seen as credible sources of such evidence. Policy decisions on issues such as poverty and mental ill health, productivity and an ageing population, waiting lists in the NHS and air travel and climate change should have a strong evidence base. However, the demand from policymakers for high-quality research evidence often outmatches the supply from researchers. This makes the best available evidence a valued commodity, as long as researchers can get it to the right recipients.

Researchers who want to create impact cannot simply wait in their academic office or laboratory for policy makers to come calling. They need to go where the policymakers are and they also need to know how the system works. In the UK, the parliament is not a single, unified institution that allows for simple contact and meaningful engagement. Rather, there are three main points of contact for researchers: the Select Committees, the Parliamentary Office of Science and Technology (POST) and the Parliamentary Libraries. The first of these is a valued resource for researchers for as Cleevely [14] stated, the UK government adopts up to 40% of select committee recommendations.

But this is just the first step; each of these points of contact for researchers work in different ways and has different audiences. Members of Parliament (MPs) and members of the House of Lords (Peers) rely on POST to provide them with readable overviews of research, in the form of POSTnotes. The Parliamentary Libraries conduct impartial and confidential research literature reviews for MPs and Peers. In contrast, Select Committees scrutinise government policy, and their reports are available to the general public and the media, as well as the government.

Not only must researchers be aware of these structures and how the function, they must be creative in how they engage with them. Their engagement needs to be timely and their reports need to be easily digestible. To become influential, researchers and their work must be on the radar of these networks and must be seen as credible sources of evidence that can underpin policy. In other words, researchers must be known and respected by MPs, Peers and parliamentary civil servants.

Researchers have to engage early to strengthen the likelihood of being noticed and their research results being taken up. As outlined elsewhere in this textbook, the most influential form of engagement is through co-creating research with research end users, in this case, policymakers. Therefore, researchers should involve parliamentary powerbrokers and stakeholders from conception to the design, conduct, dissemination, uptake, implementation and impact. Timing is crucial and readers will not be surprised to note that policymakers may be more susceptible to approaches from researchers during a budget cycle or an election campaign or when an international decision making summit is being planned.

Researchers must also acknowledge that policymaking is ideologically driven and be willing to accept that politicians disagree with each other. According to the Oxford Thesaurus [15], the following terms are synonymous with politician: bureaucrat, manipulator, machinator and influence peddler. In his diary, the British politician Alan Clark stated that *there are no true friends in politics. We are all sharks circling and waiting for traces of blood to appear in the water*' ([16], p 256).

In essence, politicians seek evidence to undermine the emerging policies of political rivals. Researcher should not be surprised if their study findings are criticised in public and in political debate or if the findings of other researchers are used to undermine theirs. Having resilience against such naysayers is a useful trait for those researchers who want to have impact through new policies.

Individual researchers can take a long time to breech the walls of government, where policymakers reside. Universities can facilitate this by establishing networks and bodies to bring policymakers and researchers together. One very helpful initiative is the Centre for Science and Policy (CSaP) at the University of Cambridge, UK. Since 2009, it has pioneered new ways of bringing together public policy professionals and academics to learn from each other. This is achieved by building relationships based on mutual understanding, respect and trust. The experience and diversity of this network provides fresh perspectives and critical challenges to conventional thinking. It also helps researchers from all disciplines to contribute more effectively to society.

CSaP's *modus operandi* is to arrange for officials from all parts of government to meet individual researchers to discuss problems and solutions. The benefits for researchers are that they get a chance to explain their work to an audience that they might otherwise struggle to reach and, in return, get fresh perspectives on policy issues. The benefits for policymakers are that they encounter new ideas and establish a network of researchers that they can call on later when they need such expertise. Neither side has to change the timescales of their work or the required levels of proof and evidence, what Cleevely [14] called the traditional barriers between policymaking and academia. This creates mutual respect and in some cases admiration. The lesson from CSaP is that a plethora of high-quality research reports have next to no impact without meaningful engagement with policymakers.

As alluded to in previous chapters, most researchers do not get their CV and ego boosted or rewarded financially or creatively by building networks with non-researchers outside of the academy. It is not their natural habitat. Similarly, policymakers seldom read academic papers and those that do seldom cite the papers in a policy document. Accepting this, Cleevely [14] con-

cluded that the CSaP should hire specialists such as events and operations managers and build the IT systems needed to identify people and run meetings. Not only was that more efficient and had lower costs, it allowed people to do what they were best suited for and more comfortable with.

Another useful resource worth checking out is the Universities Policy Engagement Network (UPEN) [17]. The is a community of UK universities committed to increasing the impact of research on policy. It offers a dedicated contact point for policymakers and a collective response to requests for evidence. It also organises knowledge exchange events with government, parliament and devolved bodies and identifies mechanisms to take forward specific projects. Furthermore, UPEN is developing best practice among universities in policy engagement activities and will act as a champion for this relatively new role within universities.

6.7   The Ten Commandments for Influencing Policymakers

Reflection Point 6.3 How to Access and Influence Policymakers
Researchers have got what policymakers need and want but they may not yet have convinced policymakers of this because not all researchers have convinced themselves. In the Times Higher Education, Diana Beech [18] identified what she referred to as the ten commandments for influencing policymakers. These can usefully be applied to how researchers can best work with policy makers to generate research impact.

6.7.1   Get to Know the People Who Really Matter

This is based on the adage that politicians come and go, but civil servants are there for a long time and they have long memories. Spending time trying to meet and build a relationship with ministers is hardly wasting time, but do not be surprised if 6 months later, they have moved on and the relationship building has to start again with a new minister. Civil servants also move around but less often than politicians and remember they could move to an even more important department. In essence, it is officials who provide continuity and stability in the research policy relationship. Do not make the mistake of falling out with civil servants simply because you have a good relationship with politicians.

6.7.2   Do not Just Criticise, Offer Solutions

Most policies can be picked apart, especially if the perspective is from the political opposition. Policymakers realise this but do not welcome researchers criticising what they have spent months getting through the various parliamentary committees. In such situations, policymakers welcome solutions not brickbats—they can get the latter in abundance from their political opponents. Beech [18] suggested helping them by being proactive and keeping ideas short, simple and jargon-free.

6.7.3   Give Policymakers a Strong Narrative

As can be seen from the various sources of information that MPs and Peers have available to them, policymakers are rarely short of statistics. What they often lack are robust qualitative narratives, as are seen in well-crafted impact case studies. Researchers have the luxury of conducting structured interviews or focus groups where they encounter rich stories, and these are a powerful way for politicians to get their message across.

6.7.4   Use Social Media Sparingly

In a previous section, I discussed the importance of altmetrics in the creation of a presence in social media. Using an MPs' or a Peers' Twitter handle, Facebook profile or LinkedIn profile can be a good way for a researcher to get their research findings on a policymaker's radar. But politicians get hundreds of social media messages each day from constituents on a range of issues. If researchers are seen to be adding to this burden without offering solutions, they can come across as annoying self-publicists.

6.7.5   Use Ministerial Priorities as a Hook

Politicians have hobbies, interests and initiatives, about which they care passionately. These are often in the public domain and can be unearthed by a few Google searches, a trawl of their Facebook pages, or a perusal of their past speeches in Hansard. Researchers should take time to find out what these interests are and use them in tailoring their approach. Human nature tells us that people are more likely to listen to your message if you frame it around something they care about personally. Politicians are no different.

6.7.6   Keep Politics Out of It

At the present time, Covid-19 and Brexit are hot political topics. Researchers are often asked by the media for their views on such issues. Do not expect to criticise policies in public and then meet with the politicians to discuss how your research can influence policy. Researchers will not ingratiate themselves if they publicly criticise a politician's politics, party or leader. The correct approach is to appear professional and constructive. Civil servants will be aware of researchers who say different things to different political parties to gain favour. Social policy academics are frequently panellists on political television programmes. They retain that regular paid media slot by challenging policies and politicians and being controversial. While this behaviour will increase the reach of the researcher's viewpoints, it will seldom be significant as it is not likely to win many friends in policymaking circles.

6.7.7 When Ministers Change, Start Again

I stated above that politicians come and go. One week, lobbyists are queuing up outside their constituency office to speak to them, the next week they are out of office, and the same lobbyists would not cross the street to greet them. This is the reality of political careers. As Enoch Powell (1912–1998) famously stated, '*all political careers end in failure*'. Therefore, do not assume that because a minister has agreed to read your research report, that a new minister will do so if the former incumbent loses office. You will need to start again; as Beech [18] noted, each minister starts afresh with a clean diary. Furthermore, they may or may not have been friends with their predecessor, so it is better not to have any political opinion of the former's successes or failings.

6.7.8 Treat Returning Ministers Like New Ministers

All ministers have independent Special Advisors (SPADS) whose job is to advise the minister and protect them from making a *faux pas*. It is good practice to get to know these SPADS and build a trusting relationship with them. Occasionally, ministers can get reappointed after they have been out of office for a period. Researchers should not take it for granted that the minister will still have the same contact details or will still be serviced by the same SPAD. New relationships may have to be built and new contact details exchanged.

6.7.9 Do Not Overlook the Power of Constituency MPs

In politics there are ministers and there are jobbing MPs working out of remote constituency offices. Three things to remember: (1) it is easier to gain access to a constituency MP than a minister, (2) a constituency MP may get a researcher access to a minister or pass a message on and (3) constituency MPs may become ministers one

day, and they will remember you if you had been helpful to them previously. All powerful political leaders started off their political career at the bottom; if a researcher's results helped them create policy that made a difference and got them promoted in their party, they will be indebted and more willing to help that individual.

6.7.10 Above All, Be Consistent

Beech [18] stressed that if researchers want policy makers to take their research seriously, the worst thing they can do is to say one thing and then do another. For example, it is not good to push research on policies to reduce global warming if the minister knows a researcher uses international air travel consistently to speak at global conferences. Such inconsistency undermines the research evidence and the significance of any impact.

In essence, Beech's ten commandments appear to be common sense. They focus on building relationships and avoiding pitfalls that will undermine trust. It is difficult for researchers to access ministers and even more difficult to influence them to create new research-informed policy. To ignore these commandments makes it almost impossible (see Appendix D).

6.8 A Communications Toolkit for Healthcare Impact

As the research community continues to produce a wealth of rich data and findings, both researchers and funders share a collective responsibility to get high-quality, robust information out to policymakers in order to bring about positive change. Thanks to advances in technology, emerging methodologies and innovative new concepts, we live in an exciting age of research unparalleled in terms of both quality and scope. At the same time, we have increased opportunities to target a wider range of audiences through a growing array of communication channels. As alluded to continually in this book, effective communication and dissemination of research are key to achieving impact. To this end, the Health Foundation worked with researchers and funders to develop a new free online communications tool to generate impact [19].

The toolkit was designed to help researchers increase the influence and impact of their research findings in health care. It does this through engaging with them at the start of their project to help them write a comprehensive communications strategy and plan. It identifies and involves key audiences so that they are connected and ready to actively receive findings throughout a project's lifespan, helping those findings gain traction.

The toolkit has three learning sections:

Section 1: Planning for Impact

This section helps researchers to plan their communications activity and focus on making impact. It deals with issues such as using strategic communications planning to increase impact, identifying and prioritising audiences, and choosing the right communications channels.

Section 2: Communicating Your Research Results

This section assists researchers to adapt and present their findings for different audiences. It focuses on how to create messages, how to effectively present research findings and how to turn planning into action.

Section 3: Extending Influence and Widening Impact

This section enables researchers to understand how to engage three of the key audiences for research dissemination and achieve impact on policy and practice. It does this through teaching them how to demonstrate impact through communications activity, how to influence a policy audience, how to engage a practice audience and how to communicate with the public.

The toolkit (see Table 6.1) has a useful free guide to demonstrating impact through networking and communications using what it refers to as Outputs, Outtakes and Outcomes.

By using such approaches to track the impact of their engagement with the public or policymakers, researchers can determine the benefit, value and influence of their work. However, gathering qualitative and quantitative impact indicators for some studies may not be easy due to the logistics involved and as outlined in the introduction, this is not the natural habitat for researchers. In addition, it can also be very difficult to isolate the specific contribution that communicating the research has had on changes in policy, practice or behaviour [19]. This goes some way to explaining why REF expert panel assessors do not see many impact case studies based on public

Table 6.1 Impact through communication and networking [19]

		Outputs	Outtakes	Outcomes
Indicators		Message to target audience	Responses and reactions of target audience	The effect (Impact) on the target audience
Quantitative indicators		• Published articles • Events held and type and number of attendees • Media articles or broadcasts achieved and potential audience size • Social media posts or tweets • Website click-throughs	• Audience members requesting or downloading information • People liking, sharing or commenting on social media • Time visitors spend on web page	• Changed attitude or perception of target audience • People changing behaviour and the associated impact • People taking an action such as registering for an activity
Qualitative indicators		• Event feedback forms showing positive comments on the event • Messages about the research in the media • Tone of media coverage	• People's ability to recall content showing awareness • Written communication from stakeholders welcoming the study • Journalists call for policy change as a result of the research • A member of a professional body discusses the research in a conference to their networks	• Research referenced in a policy paper showings its influence • Endorsement by an opinion former that influences policy change • A professional society changes guidance in response to the research

engagement. It may also explain why universities have a risk aversion to submitting such case studies for assessment in the REF.

6.9 Research Methods the Encourage Impact

Reflection Point 6.4 Embedding Impact Creation into the Research Design
Are there specific research designs and methods that enable impact generation and how do they achieve this?

Some research methods lend themselves better to public engagement than others, and because of this, they have a better chance of bringing about research impact. Engaging the public in research has become more prevalent in recent years. This might take the shape of citizen science or personal and public involvement (PPI) in research. It could be argued that including PPI in projects ensures that research will be better targeted to what society wants and needs. Erinma Ochu, a public engagement fellow at the Wellcome Trust, stated that an increase in citizen science programmes about the environment has led to more public interest in environmental issues [20]. If we translate that approach to health research, we might see people getting more invested in their own health care. In addition, sometimes the public, while they may not see the data pattern that academics see, they might perceive something a little different that has societal benefit.

For some researchers engaging in participatory, bottom-up research approaches are their preferred methodology [21]. Three increasingly popular phrases that have recently been introduced into our lexicon are 'co-design', 'co-production' and 'co-creation'. It places people at the centre of decision-making and aims to connect people together in representative networks so that they can meaningfully influence, shape and participate as real partners in the commissioning, planning, delivery and evaluation of services. In practice, co-production involves partnering with people from the start to the end of any change that affects them. It works best when people are empowered to influence decision-making for impact to occur.

The participatory research approach encapsulates the concepts of co-design, co-production, and co-creation. It is an approach to research in communities that emphasises participation and action. It seeks to understand the world by trying to change it, collaboratively. Within such studies, everyone who has a stake in the intervention has a voice, either in person or by representation. Staff of the organisation that will run it, members of the target population, community officials, interested citizens and people from involved agencies, schools and other institutions all should be invited to the table. Such a research method embeds public engagement at its core and can help to demonstrate the impact of the research throughout all the many different partners.

Readers will agree that there is a greater chance that external stakeholders will change their views and behaviour if they are involved as active researchers themselves. Participatory research has many labels; it is often termed Participatory Action Research (PAR), Community-Based Study, Co-operative Enquiry, Action Science, Real World Research and Action Learning. However, some authors prefer to see them as distinct, though related methodologies. According to Peter Reason [22], action research seeks to contribute directly to the flourishing of individuals, their communities and the ecosystems of which they are part. Its aim is to open communicative spaces where people can come together in open dialogue to address issues of concern and to engage in cycles of action and reflection. Such cycles of action are precursors to research impact.

For Koshy et al. [23], action research is mostly used in healthcare research. The community of enquiry may be composed of health professionals and patients or service users. This reflects a philosophy of 'research with' rather than 'research on' or 'research to' approaches. Multidisciplinary teams are also often involved. The key is that all participating researchers should ideally be involved in the process of data collection, data analysis, planning and implementing action, and validating evidence and critical reflection, before applying the findings. This leads to improving their own practice or the effectiveness of the system within which they work [23]. This often leads to research impact simply because all stakeholders have 'skin in the game'.

6.10 Open Science and Engagement for Impact

Open science is a relatively new movement that has strong links with public engagement for impact. Put simply, it makes research easily accessible to the general public, to industry, businesses and policymakers. Vicente-Saez and Martinez-Fuentes [24] perceived it as a transparent initiative ensuring that knowledge is shared and developed through collaborative networks. It is best understood though the term 'open access', which encourages the communication and sharing of scientific knowledge. Traditionally, people who wanted to read a research publication had to make a payment subscription to the journal or contact the author to ask for a copy from a limited supply of offprints. This reflected what may be described as 'closed science' and the business interests of publishing houses. Even research grant awarding bodies could not get immediate access to the publications emanating from the very studies they funded.

Open access changed all this; it was initiated by calls from funding organisations and government bodies to ensure that research findings could be shared free with end users as soon as possible. Researchers can make their work immediately available if they pay an author charge up front. This varied from hundreds to thousands of pounds, and the system is called Gold Open Access. Alternatively, researchers can place their published papers on a university repository, and these can be accessed after an agreed embargoed

period of time. Because there are no author costs, this is known as Green Open Access.

It makes sense that if research findings are available freely to the general public, industry, businesses and policymakers as soon as they are published, then the knowledge is more quickly disseminated and more easily assimilated. In theory, this means that uptake of the findings can be enhanced, and they can be implemented faster. During the Covid-19 pandemic, members of the public and policymakers were hungry for knowledge on everything from available vaccines to whether or not they should wear facemasks in public. Not only did they crave such research findings, they wanted them immediately! Open science was crucial in this process and speeded up the dissemination, uptake, implementation and impact of research results. The communication of research through open science has the potential to increase public trust and confidence in researchers and makes it more likely that impact will be created.

6.11 Examples of Public Engagement's Impact on Policy and Society

The REF guidelines produced by Research England [25] give examples of various types of research impact and their related indicators for reach and significance. I have extracted those that signify public engagement and policy change in Table 6.2.

6.12 Summary

This chapter deals with the generation of impact through public engagement and through influencing policy makers. The reasons why universities are reluctant to submit such impact case studies to the REF are explored. The cause is mainly around reach and significance. The former is easily achieved and assessed in most public engagement activities but whether there are any significant benefits is less easily evidenced. Strategies for engaging with policymakers were

Table 6.2 Examples of public engagement and policy impact with related evidence of reach and significance

Areas of impact	Types of impact	Reach and significance indicators
Impact on social welfare where the beneficiaries include individuals, groups of individuals, organisations or communities whose rights, duties, behaviours, opportunities, inclusion, quality of life and other activity have been influenced	• Engagement with research has enhanced policy and practice for securing poverty alleviation	• Documented evidence of changes to social policy
Impacts on public policy, law and services where the beneficiaries are usually government, non-governmental organisations (NGOs), charities and public sector organisations and society, either as a whole or groups of individuals in society, through the implementation or non-implementation of policies, systems or reforms	• Policy debate has been stimulated or informed by research evidence, which may have led to confirmation of policy, change in policy direction, implementation or withdrawal of policy • A policy has been implemented (including those realised through changes to legislation) or the delivery of a public service has changed • (Sections of) the public have benefited from public service improvements • The work of an NGO, charitable or other organisation has been influenced by the research • Policy decisions or changes to legislation, regulations or guidelines have been informed by research evidence • In delivering a public service, a new technology or process has been adopted or an existing technology or process improved • The quality, accessibility, acceptability or cost-effectiveness of a public service has been improved • Risks to the security of nation states have been reduced	• Documented evidence of use in policy debate (e.g. at a parliamentary Select Committee, material produced by NGOs) • Citation in a public discussion, consultation document or judgement • Evidence of citation in policy, regulatory, strategy, practice or other documents • Direct citations of research in parliamentary publications such as Hansard, committee reports, evidence submissions or briefings • Acknowledgements to researchers on webpages, in reports or briefings • Evidence of influence on a debate in public policy and practice through membership of or distinctive contributions to expert panels and policy committees or advice to government (at local, national or international level) • Quantitative indicators or statistics on the numbers of attendees or participants at a research event, or website analytics for online briefings
Impacts on understanding, learning and participation where the beneficiaries are individuals, communities and organisations whose awareness, understanding or participation	• Enhanced cultural understanding of issues and phenomena; shaping or informing public attitudes and values • Public interest and engagement in research has been stimulated through, for example the enhancement of science education in schools	• Many organisations use the Generic Learning Outcomes (GLO) to evaluate impacts on knowledge and understanding

presented, and they too can easily show reach but significance can be absent or not measurable. Some research methods lend themselves to the generation of impact simply because their phi-losophy is based on close working relationships with end users of research. Participatory Action Research is one such approach. Finally, the recently introduction of open science means that dissemination of research findings to external stakeholders is speeded up considerably and this can lead to early adoption of results and the creation of impact. The next chapter deals with evidence-informed practice and its links to research impact. The principles can be extrapolated to evidence-informed policymaking, and hence, this chapter forms the basis for that relationship.

References

1. Chiyson AS. The sagacity of sage. Living with excellence. New York, NY: Seaburn; 2008. ISBN-10: 1592321534.
2. Finkle A. Evidence and integrity. Science meets parliament 2018, Canberra. Opening Address; 2018. https://www.chiefscientist.gov.au/sites/default/files/Chief-Scientist-Science-meets-Parliament.pdf.
3. KEF. Knowledge exchange framework. Research England. 2020. https://re.ukri.org/knowledge-exchange/knowledge-exchange-framework/.
4. Womersley J. Scientists are getting drawn into messy, polarised debates'. 2020. https://www.researchprofessional.com/0/rr/news/europe/views-of-europe/2020/6/-Exposure-to-politics-is-making-science-worse-.html?utm_medium=email&utm_source=rpMailing&utm_campaign=personalNewsDailyUpdate_2020-06-03#sthash.GvtsifeS.dpuf.
5. Aksoy CG, Eichengreen B, Saka O. Revenge of the experts: will COVID 19 renew or diminish public trust in science? SRC discussion paper no 96. London: SRC; 2020. http://www.systemicrisk.ac.uk/sites/default/files/downloads/publications/dp-96_0.pdf ISSN2054-538X.
6. Halpern M. Italian scientists jailed for failing to predict earthquake. Cambridge, MA: Union of Concerned Scientists; 2012. https://blog.ucsusa.org/michael-halpern/italian-scientists-jailed-for-failing-to-predict-earthquake.
7. NCCPE. National Co-ordinating Centre for Public Engagement. 2020. https://www.publicengagement.ac.uk/about-engagement.
8. Priem J. Altmetrics. 2020. https://www.researchgate.net/profile/Jason_Priem.
9. Fenner M. Altmetrics and other novel measures for scientific impact. 2015. http://book.openingscience.org/vision/altmetrics.html.
10. Bornmann L, Haunschild R, Adams J. Do altmetrics assess societal impact in a comparable way to case studies? An empirical test of the convergent validity of altmetrics based on data from the UK Research Excellence Framework; 2018. https://arxiv.org/ftp/arxiv/papers/1807/1807.03977.pdf.
11. Loach T, Adams J, Szomszor M. Digital research report: the societal and economic impacts of academic research—international perspectives on good practice and managing evidence. 2016. doi:10.6084/m9.figshare.3117928.v2.
12. Adams J, Bornmann L, Haunschild R. Excellence is useful. Research Fortnight 18 Apr; 2019. https://www.researchprofessional.com/0/rr/news/europe/views-of-europe/2019/4/Excellence-is-useful.html?utm_medium=email&utm_source=rpMailing&utm_campaign=personalNewsDailyUpdate_2019-04-18#sthash.ceMccvrH.dpuf.
13. Lexico. Lexico US dictionary; 2020. https://www.lexico.com/en/definition/policy.
14. Cleevely D. 11 Jun 2018 Only connect- how to help academics influence policy; 2018. https://www.researchprofessional.com/0/rr/news/uk/views-of-the-uk/2018/6/Only-connect-how-to-help-academics-influence-policy.html?utm_medium=email&utm_source=rpMailing&utm_campaign=personalNewsDailyUpdate_2018-06-11#sthash.r2P1JPSX.dpuf.
15. Oxford Thesaurus. Oxford dictionary and thesaurus. Oxford: Oxford Lanuguages; 2007.
16. Clark A. Dairies: in power 1983–1992. London: Weidenfeld and Nicholson; 2003.
17. UPEN. Universities Policy Engagement Network. 2020. https://www.upen.ac.uk/.
18. Beech D. Ten commandments for influencing policymakers in turbulent times. The Times Higher Education; 2019. https://www.timeshighereducation.com/opinion/ten-commandments-influencing-policy-makers-turbulent-times.
19. The Health Foundation. Communicating your research – a toolkit help increase influence and impact in health and health care. 2017. https://www.health.org.uk/publications/communicating-your-research-a-toolkit.
20. Ochu E. Citizen social science deepens the human and relational aspects of the social scientific method. LSE blog; 2014. https://blogs.lse.ac.uk/impactofsocialsciences/2014/02/27/citizen-social-science-human-method/.
21. Fahy F. Participatory action research in environmental and ecological studies. In: International encyclopedia of the social & behavioral sciences. 2nd ed. London: Elsevier; 2015. ISBN 978-0-08-097087-52015.
22. Reason P. Action research. Encyclopaedia Britannica. 2020. https://www.britannica.com/topic/action-research.
23. Koshy V, et al. Action research. New York, NY: Sage Publications; 2010. https://www.sagepub.com/sites/default/files/upm-binaries/36584_01_Koshy_et_al_Ch_01.pdf.

24. Vicente-Saez R, Martinez-Fuentes C. Open science now: a systematic literature review for an integrated definition. J Business Res. 2018;88:428–36. https://doi.org/10.1016/j.jbusres.2017.12.043.

25. Research England. The research excellence framework. 2020. https://re.ukri.org/research/research-excellence-framework-ref/.

Research Impact: The Link to Evidence-Informed Practice

'The child in the womb of his mother looks from one end of the world to the other and knows all the teaching, but the instant he comes in contact with the air of earth, an angel strikes him on the mouth and he forgets everything'.

(Rodkinson [1])

7.1 Introduction

It can be seen by the graphs in Chap. 8 that a large number of research impact case studies submitted in REF 2014 in health science focused on improving clinical practice and improving the scientific basis for patient care and treatment. It could be argued that the concepts 'research impact' and 'evidence-informed practice' are the same. There are of course some obvious similarities; impact requires high-quality research to underpin it, as does evidence-informed practice. However, I will argue that they are not the same and that evidence-informed practice may be an important precursor to research impact. Furthermore, I will show that evidence-informed practice is not the same as research-informed practice. Nonetheless, let me commence with an examination of the use of evidence-informed practice.

The extract from the Talmud at the start of this chapter seems to indicate that at one stage we had all the evidence we needed to solve our global problems but on being born, we lost it. As a useful metaphor, researchers have spent generations attempting to reclaim and implement some of what the Angel took from us. Researchers con-

tinue the quest for the best available evidence to drive changes and benefits for humankind—in other words, to have impact.

Consider the following scenario: a doctor goes out to lunch with some friends who do not work in health care. They ask her what is new in her field. She mentions that evidence-informed practice is a popular phenomenon. When they enquire as to what this means, she says that it involves providing patients with care and treatment that is underpinned by the most up-to-date research. They look surprised and ask her if this is not something that health professionals have always done!

Why should they be surprised? Well today, someone somewhere is receiving a service or an intervention that is out of date or that is not underpinned by sound evidence. We should be very concerned about this. Distributive justice dictates that everyone has an unqualified right to the very best health care. This underpins clear legal and moral rights, such as to be treated in the best possible way within available resources.

The parallel with research impact is obvious. Throughout this book, I have employed the synonyms benefit and change to explain research impact. These are also the goals of evidence-

H. P. McKenna, *Research Impact*, https://doi.org/10.1007/978-3-030-57028-6_7

informed practice. Both want to stop interventions that do more harm than good and start interventions that do more good than harm. I will argue later that in this regard research impact goes further than evidence-informed practice.

7.2   Some Background

It is generally agreed that as a movement, evidence-informed practice was 'kick started' by a lecture given by Archie Cochrane, of Cochrane Review fame. He was a doctor and epidemiologist. In 1972 he aroused a lot of interest by pointing out that many decisions about health are made without up-to-date evidence for the care and treatments used, the very antithesis of research impact.

Cochrane's [2] lecture was a culmination of concerns he had expressed over many years. It was motivated originally by his experiences as a prisoner of war during World War Two. He noted with great regret that people were dying because of the medical attention they received, rather than the lack of it. Reflecting back, Cochrane stated:

> I would gladly have sacrificed my freedom for a little knowledge. I had never heard then of "Randomised Controlled Trials", but I knew there was no real evidence that anything we had to offer had any effect ... and I was afraid that I shortened the lives of some of my friends by unnecessary intervention [3].

Here Cochrane admits that because of a lack of research, some of his interventions had a negative rather than a positive impact on patients. It represents an apt example of how high-quality underpinning research is a requirement for positive impact. Without research evidence, clinicians are working in the dark and the result is that impacts on patient care and treatment become a hit and miss affair.

Reflection Point 7.1 The Importance of Terminology

Consider the terms evidence-based practice, practice-based evidence and evidence-informed practice. Which do you prefer and why?

In 1992, 20 years after Cochrane's lecture, David Sackett coined the term evidence-based medicine [4]. Two years later, the expression evidence-based practice emerged. At this juncture, I should add that I am troubled by these terms. Evidence-based practice and evidence-based medicine give the impression that clinicians are non-thinking automatons who follow unquestionably the directives of researchers. But from my perspective, research results should be used to inform practice not to dictate it. This is why, I prefer the term evidence-informed practice; whenever possible, it will be the phrase I used in this chapter. But, regardless of terminology, it is a good idea to explore what it is and why we want it!

Appleby et al. [5] stated that evidence-informed practice was

> A shift in the culture of health care provision away from basing decisions on opinion, past practice and precedent toward making more use of research evidence to guide clinical decision making.

This definition is firmly linked to research impact. It implies that decisions should be made based on rigorous underpinning research. Nonetheless, I would argue that it is not a definition of research impact; rather it is one step removed. If we revisit the research continuum, outlined in Chap. 1, we can see this more clearly. Obtain a Research Grant → Conduct the Research → Disseminate the Findings → **Uptake → Implementation** → Impact. Readers will agree that evidence-informed practice fits within the uptake and implementation stages but is one step removed from research impact. In other words, research impact is the end result of evidence-informed practice, or should be!

Let us examine another popular definition of evidence-informed practice. DiCenso et al. [6] put forward a less rigid and almost contradictory definition to that of Appleby.

> A process by which clinicians make clinical decisions using the best available research evidence,

their clinical expertise and patient preferences in the context of available resources.

Look at these definitions carefully; I want you to note that neither of them refers specifically to research impact or indeed any outcome—a familiar pattern in definitions of evidence-informed practice. Rather, each concentrates on the 'thinking and doing' aspects of practice, suggesting that the term evidence-informed practice relates specifically to uptake and implementation, not impact. The fact that these processes should be linked with positive impact is not a matter for explicit consideration by these authors. Therefore, my first key message for readers is that the best available evidence to underpin practice must be continually evaluated to ensure that it takes that final step to achieving impact. It is not beyond the realm of possibility that some evidence-informed decisions or practices do not change anything. I will return to this theme below when I compare the concepts 'certainty' with 'agreement'.

Another point to notice about these definitions is that what DeCenso et al. would identify as evidence would not be perceived as such by Appleby et al. From the latter's perspective, evidence is reliant on the existence of research findings. In contrast, DeCenso stated that clinical expertise and patient preferences are also sources of evidence. In the context of the REF, the latter definition would not satisfy the criteria that impact must be underpinned by quality research; expertise and preferences would not count. An impact case study built on such evidence would not meet the 2 star quality threshold and would be rated unclassified.

This apparent contradiction between these two definitions may be explained by what Muir Gray [7] called the Hierarchy of Evidence (see Table 7.1).

You will notice that the top four levels describe accepted research designs, and any one of them could be used to generate underpinning research for impact. Level V has much in common with DeCenso's definition and, as alluded to above, would not be currently acceptable by expert panel assessors in REF. This may of course change in future REFs as the definition of research broadens to encapsulate other types of outputs. In fact, the Stern Report [8] recommended that evidence of research underpinning impact should go beyond the presentation of research papers.

Table 7.1 The hierarchy of evidence [7]

Level I	Meta-analysis of a series of randomised controlled trials
Level II	At least one well-designed randomised controlled trial
Level III	At least one controlled study without randomisation
Level IV	Well-designed non-experimental studies
Level V	Case reports, clinical examples, opinion of experts

Let me explore this a little further; physicians with many years' experience may use their clinical expertise and/or the case reports of patients they have treated to decide on a healthcare intervention. It is possible that the patients respond positively to the intervention and their healthcare improves. Using the synonyms of change and benefit here, there is no doubt that positive impact was achieved and reach and significance may be claimed. However, under the current REF rules, such impact would be discounted. This is not surprising; after all, the REF is an exercise focused on research quality, not the quality of expert opinion!

The type of understanding encapsulated by opinion and clinical expertise has been referred to as tacit knowledge or what Michael Polanyi, a Nobel prize-winning physical chemist called 'Personal Knowledge' [9]. His wide-ranging research in physical science reflects the highest scientific investigations into chemical kinetics, X-ray diffraction and adsorption of gases. But Polanyi claimed that all knowledge claims, including those emanating from scientific research, rely on personal judgements. To him, Personal Knowledge is the ability to achieve something, without necessarily being able to articulate why it happened.

Reflection Point 7.2 What It Means to Be an Expert
Consider three occupations or professions where knowledge and skills are honed to perfection over a number of years and where an activity can be undertaken expertly almost without thinking. Such activities can

have impact but what type of knowledge are they based on, if not research?

In her textbook *From Novice to Expert* (1984), Patricia Benner recognised that as clinicians travelled along the continuum from novice to expert, they gained knowledge and skills ('know how'), without ever learning the theory or the science ('know that'). She based her work on the Dreyfus Model of Skill Acquisition [10]. Stuart and Hubert Dreyfus observed chess players, air force pilots, army commanders and tank drivers. Their research findings led them to believe that learning was experiential (learning through experience) as well as situation-based. They also maintained that a learner had to pass through five very distinct stages, from novice to expert. They noted than an experienced pilot can look at the instruments in an aircraft in a holistic way—seeing the whole ensemble rather than the individual parts.

Benner found similar parallels in nursing, where improved practice depended on experience and science, and developing those skills was a long and progressive process. As with the Dreyfus brothers, she identified five stages that practitioners pass through on the route to the development of clinical expertise. The first stage is being a **Novice**, where there is a very limited ability to predict what might happen in a particular patient situation. Signs and symptoms, such as change in mental status, can only be recognized after a novice clinician has had experience with patients with similar symptoms. The next stage is **Advanced Beginner**, where clinicians have had more experiences that enable them to recognize recurrent, meaningful components of a situation. They have the knowledge and the know-how but not enough in-depth experience.

The next stage is being **Competent**; here the clinicians lack the speed and flexibility of proficient practitioners, but they recognise the patterns and nature of clinical situations more quickly and accurately than advanced beginners.

The fourth stage is being **Proficient**, where clinicians are capable of seeing situations as 'wholes' rather than parts. The final stage is being an **Expert**; here individuals no longer rely solely on rules to guide their actions. They have an intuitive grasp of the situation based on their deep knowledge, skills and experience.

There are numerous examples of where experienced clinicians were able to predict a problem with a patient before it occurred. When asked how they knew what was going to happen, the common response is 'I just knew'. Readers will agree that such intuitive knowledge can be impactful and make a real difference, but no university is going to risk submitting such an impact case study in the REF. Perhaps if it could be measured in some way, it might be more acceptable, but this raises other issues.

Even though he was trained as a physical scientist, Michael Polanyi was very critical of **Galileo Galilei** who famously stated:

Count what is countable, measure what is measurable and what is not measurable—make measurable (cited in [11]).

But many of the issues of importance to health care defy quantification: how do you calibrate compassion? how do you quantify a presence? how do you measure empathy? Nonetheless, from a research impact point of view, Galileo's approach would be closer to acceptability in REF than Polanyi's views. Of course, we have seen in Chap. 2 that REF impact case studies are mainly qualitative narratives, interspersed with quantitative indicators. This suggests that qualitative narratives describing personal knowing may be acceptable, if combined with quantitative indicators based on 2 star research.

To return to Archie Cochrane for a moment; he was to a large extent the instigator of the gold standard randomized controlled trial (RCT). RCTs can be good at determining cause and effect, and this is often the basis for research impact. In this regard Cochrane would be very much in the Galileo camp. However, in an almost Damascene conversion, he too realised that other non-research approaches were needed to have a positive impact on human problems [12].

'… The Germans dumped a young Soviet prisoner in my ward late one night. The ward was full, so I put him in my room as he was moribund and screaming and I did not want to wake the ward … He had obvious gross bilateral cavitation and a severe pleural rub. I thought the latter was the cause of the pain and the screaming. I had no morphia, just aspirin, which had no effect … I felt desperate … I finally instinctively sat down on the bed and took him in my arms, and the screaming stopped almost at once. He died peacefully in my arms a few hours later. It was not the pleurisy that caused the screaming but loneliness. It was a wonderful education about the care of the dying. I was ashamed of my misdiagnosis and kept the story secret'.

So over time Archie Cochrane had other views about what may or may not be an effective way to achieve an impact; it was not always achieved through the results of a RCT.

Evidence is a victim of time. What was evidence last year may not be evidence this year. At one time there was evidence that boring holes in people's skulls or using leeches were perceived as good ways of controlling some symptoms or that extracting teeth was the best way to deal with dental caries. Today, such interventions are perceived as barbaric. I have no doubt that in 50 years' time, interventions that currently create impact will be denigrated by society. No crystal ball gazing but I doubt if ECT, some major surgery and many types of cancer chemotherapy (all currently underpinned by sound research) will exist. In 1973, an editorial in the journal *Nature* backed women smoking during pregnancy on the grounds that it calmed their stress [13]. See Chap. 5 for other examples of bad impact.

This has obvious implication for research impact. It is not unusual for new research findings to overturn or replace the findings previously held as best evidence. For example, in earlier chapters, readers saw how the governments approach to Covid-19 changed from supporting herd immunity to lockdown and social distancing, once new evidence took precedence.

It is not beyond the realm of possibility that the underpinning research for an outstanding impact case study in REF 2014 is overturned by new research in some future REF exercise. This does not mean that the first impact was not out-

standing; rather, knowledge moves on. This can also explain continued impact case studies, where research results of one study often build on the research results of previous studies. So, in some cases new impacts will build on previous ones in an evolutionary manner, whereas in other cases there is no link whatsoever between one impact and a newer impact on the same topic. The next few paragraphs explores this from a theoretical perspective.

Thomas Kuhn (1922–1996) asserted that science progressed through a series of revolutionary steps. After each revolution, there is a period of 'normal science' where a particular scientific worldview (paradigm) reigns supreme and scholars accept it as a basis for knowledge and truth. Rejecting this paradigm during a period of normal science would be frowned upon by the scientific community. However, according to Kuhn, it is eventually questioned, leading to what he refers to as a 'scientific revolution'. This may be because it fails to deal adequately with some new phenomenon, or a new, more powerful paradigm has great explanatory power. As more evidence accumulates to show that the old way of thinking has outlived its usefulness, a 'paradigm shift' occurs. Kuhn maintained that paradigm shifts are not cumulative and the new paradigm is not built on the previous paradigm [14]. The new paradigm becomes the focus for a new period of normal science.

Reflection Point 7.3 Revolutionary Impacts
Identify three examples where a new research-informed practice was introduced that had no link with the practice it replaced.

One example of this would be Ptolemy's (367–282 BC) teaching that the Sun orbited the Earth. This paradigm held sway for centuries in what Kuhn would call 'normal science'. However, when Copernicus (1473–1543) challenged this with his theory that the Earth moved around the Sun, a paradigm shift took place. Other examples include Newton's theory of gravity being replaced by Einstein's theory of relativity or the contemporary focus on community care as opposed to institutional care for those with mental health problems. Paradigm shifts occurred because the old paradigms were not able to explain new experiences or solve new problems.

Translating Kuhn's theory into impact speak, I will turn once again to the Covid-19 pandemic. In this example, underpinning research showed that herd immunity was the best way to deal with the virus. This was introduced across the country and became what Kuhn would call normal science. After a period of time, its impact on the spread of the virus was questioned. Based on different research, the policy changed to one of social isolation and lockdown. This was a paradigm shift because the research underpinning it was significantly different from the research underpinning herd immunity, as was the policy and practice. This change in policy and practice leading to impact is best described as revolutionary rather than evolutionary.

Kuhn's theory might also explain the concept of new impact case studies. The REF definition of these is where new research has been conducted and/or the impact types or beneficiaries have changed. Here the impact type could have changed from an impact on culture to an impact on the economy. Similarly, the beneficiaries could have changed from actors to stock brokers. Looking at this through a Kuhnian lens, there is very little relationship between the previous impact and the new impact—a revolutionary change.

Larry Laudan [15] challenged Kuhn's view that knowledge development was a revolutionary process. Rather, he believed that knowledge was developed in an evolutionary way with new knowing being influenced by previous knowing. It is best represented by Isaac Newton who stated 'If I have seen further it is by standing on the shoulders of Giants' [16]. In other words, science builds on what went before.

This *evolutionary* view propounded by Larry Laudan also fits the concept of continuing case

studies as one research impact builds on a previous impact. This means there is significant overlap with the previous impact. More generally, new research often builds on previous studies. The example of the discovery of penicillin described in Chap. 5 is a good example of this.

In the USA, Afaf Meleis [17] challenged both Kuhn and Laudan. She argued that the revolutionary and evolutionary approaches to knowledge development are too simplistic on their own to explain the progression from one impact to another. She coined the term 'convolution' to explain how knowledge often progresses, not through evolution or revolution, but through a convolutionary series of peaks, troughs, detours, backward steps and crises. This gives the impression that knowledge development is confusing and uncoordinated. There may be some truth in this, especially for some health disciplines that are in what Kuhn [14] might describe as a pre-paradigmatic stage of development. In such a neophyte discipline, without a mature body of research, impact may progress then regress to an earlier iteration before progressing again.

This convolution approach may explain the recommendation of the Stern committee that impact is not linear [8]. Rather the pathway to research impact may be non-direct and not immediate. It can occur contemporaneously with the underpinning research, and as seen in Chap. 2, impact can occur before the research outputs underpinning the research come into the public domain.

7.3   The Drive for Certainty and Agreement in Research Impact?

Researchers reach out continually for the holy grail of certainty in the pursuit of research impact. However, the world, as with life in general, is full of uncertainties. Uncertainty about impact brings anxiety and confusion, and this means that during such times, clinicians may fall back on familiar practices and routines Table 7.2.

In Area 1 are those evidence-informed practices that have high levels of agreement, but their impact is far from certain. Most of these interventions do no real harm, but they also do no real

Table 7.2 Agreement and certainty in the generation of research impact

	Far from certainty of impact	Close to certainty of impact
Close to agreement	1	2
Far from agreement	3	4

good. One example is the multiple occasions where the same details are recorded in patients' notes. Patients can be seen clinically by doctors, nurses and allied health professionals, and they all record similar information in the records. Each of these disciplines agree with the importance of patient record keeping. Perhaps the underlying cause for the unnecessary repetition is the fear of litigation. Nonetheless, it is frustration for patients to get asked the same questions several times, and it does take up a great deal of time.

The reason may also have something to do with the ritual of clinical practise; after a consultation or an intervention, it is almost a tradition that notes must be written up. Basing practice on tradition has immense benefits for some clinicians: they feel comfortable with rituals, which are often a mechanism for keeping control in a busy clinical setting where there are unpredictable and ever-changing conditions and where staff are forever altering in numbers and qualifications. Also, routines are sometimes legitimised because they were learned from the actions of an authority figure or a trusted colleague. Regardless of their origin, rituals and routines for their own sake do not underpin research impact and are seldom research based. Once again, impacts emanating from routine practices would have no place in REF.

In Area 2 are those interventions that clinicians undertake that have high levels of agreement, and there is some certainty about their impact. They are mostly underpinned by good-quality research evidence. Examples include pre-operative visits and information giving, which reduces post-operative complications, cognitive behavioural therapy to improve functioning in patients with acute psychosis and parents' active involvement in the care of their hospitalised children. Here, undoubtedly, the interventions do more good than harm, and there is consensus on the research impact generated. These examples

could form the basis for high-scoring impact case studies in the REF.

In Area 3 are those interventions that clinicians undertake that have low levels of agreement among the profession, and their impact is far from certain. These interventions do no real harm, but it is uncertain whether or not they do any good. For example, homeopathic remedies are a multimillion pound industry. Yet there is little agreement as to whether they contribute to better health care, and there is no certainty as to their impact on peoples' health.

> **Reflection Point 7.4 Ignoring Research Informed Behaviours that Have Impact**
> Try and think of two research-informed behaviours that would have a good impact, yet are ignored by many people. These can be behaviours that should be stopped or started.

Finally, in Area 4 are those interventions that have low levels of agreement, but their impact has been shown to be certain. Examples include prophylactic aspirin to avoid blood clotting and certain cancers (see impact case study in Chap. 8), regular exercise, and eating five pieces of fruit per day (see impact case study in Chap. 8). Here we know that these interventions are research informed and do more good than harm, but yet they are not universally incorporated into our practice or lifestyle. These and other similar interventions form the basis for research impact, but they need to be mainstreamed through policy and public engagement.

I suspect readers are wondering how much of healthcare activity is in Area 2. This is difficult to estimate but the idea of healthcare being 100% research informed is probably unrealistic. It is a truism, therefore, that if clinicians were told that they could only use research evidence as a basis for their interventions, impact would be seriously curtailed. To maximise research impact, we should be aiming to increase the number of interventions in Area 2 and continue to bring the interventions in Area 4 into mainstream practice. Interventions in Areas 1 and 3 should be investigated and if they do not move into Area 2, they should be stopped.

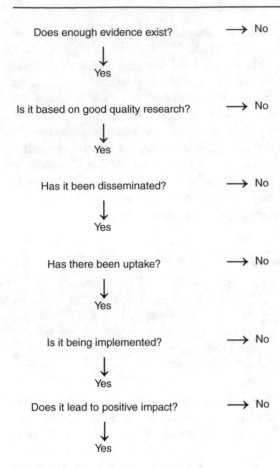

Does enough evidence exist? ⟶ No

↓

Yes

Is it based on good quality research? ⟶ No

↓

Yes

Has it been disseminated? ⟶ No

↓

Yes

Has there been uptake? ⟶ No

↓

Yes

Is it being implemented? ⟶ No

↓

Yes

Does it lead to positive impact? ⟶ No

↓

Yes

Fig. 7.1 Flowchart showing the link between evidence-informed practice and research impact

The flowchart in Fig. 7.1 links evidence-informed practice and research impact.

7.4   Research Impact: When Is Best Evidence Ignored?

Reflection Point 7.5 The Reasons for Ignoring Research Findings
In Reflection Point 7.4, you identified behaviours that people might ignore, even though the impact would be beneficial. Give three reasons why they would do this.

If I asked readers whether clinicians should use the best available evidence to achieve research impact, they would probably say yes. Who could possibly be opposed to this? But I would argue that occasionally there are some reasons why the findings from good quality research are not used to generate impact. In 1981, Jenny Hunt [18] maintained that it is because clinicians:

- Do not know about them
- Do not understand them
- Do not believe them
- Do not know how to apply them
- Are not allowed to use them

In 1978, Barbara Carper [19] identified four types of knowing in clinical practice (Empiric, Ethical, Aesthetic and Personal). I propose to change the designation from knowing to evidence. The first is '*Empiric Evidence*' and represents evidence that is **verifiable, objective, factual and research based**. This is the type of quantifiable and objective evidence seen in Area 2 in Table 7.2 or in Levels 1–4 of Muir Grey's hierarchy [7] as outlined in Table 7.1. It is the kind of evidence that underpins research in REF impact case studies. However, sometimes we can ignore this type of evidence because it is superseded by one or more of the other types of evidence.

For instance, '*Ethical Evidence*' focuses on what is right and wrong and what actions are good and bad, desirable and undesirable. For ethical reasons, some clinicians may decide not to participate in an intervention, even though the results from clinical trials or other studies note that it can have a positive impact for patients. For example, there are some clinicians who still will not participate in electroconvulsive therapy even though there is empirical research to show that it has a positive impact on patients' mental health.

Ethical Evidence may also be used to make decisions about the costs of treatment, quality-adjusted life years (QuALYs) and rationing of health care. This was a major issue for many clinicians in the recent Covid-19 pandemic. Globally, there was a shortage of ventilators, intensive care beds and personal protective equipment. Clinicians, whose job was to save lives, had to make life and death decisions on who should get access to scarce lifesaving resources. Similarly, there are occasions when it has been decided that some patients should not be resuscitated if they have a cardiac arrest. Clinically, there is *Empiric Evidence* to indicate what practice to follow. However, for ethical reasons, some clinicians may choose not to participate in such interventions.

Aesthetic Evidence and *Personal Evidence* give us the knowledge that focuses on the art of care and tacit knowledge, what Polanyi [9] called personal knowing and what Benner [20] referred to as expertise. Armed with these types of evidence, clinicians may ignore *Empirical Evidence*. For instance, there are many research-based scales that are used to assess and predict patients' discharge from acute care, risk of aggression, or suicide risk. But clinical judgement, based on experience, intuition and knowing the patient may mean that some senior clinicians decide to follow their instinct and ignore such evidence-informed measures.

Therefore. there are different types of evidence, and all have an influence on impact. While *Empiric Evidence* is the basis for most impact case studies, depending on circumstances, other types of evidence are legitimate and can also generate positive impact. Take the example of the *Empiric Evidence* that forms the basis of clinical guidelines on the mobilising of patients post-operatively. However, based on *Personal Evidence,* an experienced clinician may intuitively know that a particular patient is not ready for full mobilising. In this case, the impact based on her tacit knowledge may be better than that generated by the Empiric Evidence.

7.5   Researchers: Their Role in Encouraging or Discouraging Impact

Several of the obstacles to the use of evidence to achieve impact has to do with researchers. A research study found that clinicians did not achieve impact because of barriers to the implementation of research evidence [21]. This was due to their inability to understand statistical findings, the confusion that arises through conflicting research results (e.g. Here Immunity Vs Lockdown) and the use of too much research jargon. Perhaps, unsurprisingly they complained of the overwhelming amounts of published research papers. This latter issue is not new and is illustrated wonderfully by a building metaphor used almost 40 years ago by Raulin [22]. Let us suppose that the 'builders' (clinicians) depend upon 'brickmakers' (researchers) to produce usable bricks (research papers) so that they can make edifices (research impact). Bashford and Slevin [23] describes Raulin's fable as follows:

> And so it happened that the land became flooded with bricks. It became necessary to organise more and more storage places, called journals... in all of this the brick makers retained their pride and skill and the bricks were of the very best quality. But production was ahead of demand and...it became difficult for builders to find the proper bricks for a task because one had to hunt among so many.... It became difficult to complete a useful edifice because, as soon as the foundations were discernible, they were buried under an avalanche of random bricks. And, saddest of all, sometimes no effort was made to maintain the distinction between a pile of bricks and a true edifice.

Therefore, if we are not careful, impact can be delayed because of the plethora of evidence-based guidelines, protocols and research reports. This has the potential to alienate clinicians from researchers and disrupt the engagement that is crucial for impact to occur.

7.6　Summary

No clinician would deny that sound research evidence should be an integral part of achieving research impact. I will summarise the ten key messages emanating from this chapter:

1. Evidence-informed practice is not impact, yet it is a necessary antecedent to research impact.
2. Evidence-informed practice is really about uptake and implementation, and the end result may not be a positive impact.
3. Tacit knowing and expert experience are seen as evidence but are not a legitimate procurer to research impact.
4. There are many instances where clinicians use evidence-informed practice to achieve outstanding research impact.
5. People in need of health care have a legal and moral right to be cared for and treated so that the best impact can be achieved within available resources.
6. Ethical and Personal evidence can on occasions achieve impact through ignoring empiric (research) evidence.
7. The existence of the best available evidence is not enough—it has to be used and its impact evaluated.
8. Researchers must present their research reports in such a way that does not overwhelm or confuse clinical staff.
9. Archie Cochrane changed his views on the RCT being the underpinning basis for some impacts.
10. Interventions have the greatest impact when there is agreement and certainty on their benefits.

While the ability to produce research evidence is restricted to a small number of individuals in most professions, the knowledge of how to search for it, assess it, disseminate it, apply it in practice and assess its impact must be a major part of the mind set for every clinician. The mere existence of evidence cannot bring about research impact; it has to be used.

This chapter has shown that research-informed practice is not the same as evidence-informed practice. In other words, research is evidence, but evidence is not necessarily research. Furthermore, what is and is not evidence is fluid and relies as much on timing and choice as it does on methodology. The rule of thumb should be that it is not the best possible evidence that is required, rather it is the best evidence available at a particular time for a specific patient in a specific situation. This means that in the absence of high-quality research findings, in some situations, the patient's preference may lead to the best impact while in others it may be the results of a randomised controlled trial. We simply have to accept that as this juncture, the former type of evidence would not be acceptable in REF.

After reading this chapter, you might be forgiven for thinking that everything is evidence in one form or another. However, evidence-informed practice eradicates ritualistic, routine and traditional behaviours and ungrounded opinions as a basis for clinical impact. It highlights the importance of consensus among recognised experts, confirmed experiences and patient accounts as well as research findings and quality improvement data.

Alvin Toffler [24] wrote,

> The illiterate of the 21st century will not be those who cannot read and write, but those who cannot learn, unlearn, and relearn.

References

1. Rodkinson ML. The Babylonian Talmud. Volumes 1–10; 1918. https://www.jewishvirtuallibrary.org/jsource/Judaism/FullTalmud.pdf.
2. Cochrane A. Effectiveness and efficiency: random reflections on health services. Report on randomised controlled trials (RCTs). London: The Nuffield Trust; 1972. ISBN: 0900574178 https://www.nuffieldtrust.org.uk/research/effectiveness-and-efficiency-random-reflections-on-health-services.
3. Cochrane AL. Sickness in Salonica: my first, worst, and most successful clinical trial. Br Med J (Clin Res Ed). 1984;289(6460):1726–7. https://doi.org/10.1136/bmj.289.6460.1726. PMC 1444794. PMID 6440622.
4. Sackett DL, Rosenberg WM. The need for evidence-based medicine. J R Soc Med 1995. 1982;88(11):620–4. PMID: 8544145.

5. Appleby J, Walshe K, Ham C. Acting on the evidence, Research paper 17. London: NAHAT; 1995.

6. DiCenso A, Cullum N, Ciliska D. Implementing evidence-based nursing: some misconceptions. Evid Based Nurs. 1998;1(2) https://doi.org/10.1136/ebn.1.2.38.

7. Muir Gray JA. Evidence based healthcare: how to make health policy and management decisions. New York: Churchill Livingstone; 1997.

8. Stern N. Building on success and learning from experience an independent review of the research excellence framework. London: Department of Business, Energy and Industrial Strategy; 2016. https://assets.publishing.service.gov.uk/government/uploads/system/uploads/attachment_data/file/541338/ind-16-9-ref-stern-review.pdf.

9. Polanyi M. The tacit dimension. Chicago, IL: University of Chicago Press; 1966. ISBN 978-0-226-67298-4. OCLC 262429494.

10. Dreyfus SE, Dreyfus HL. A five-stage model of the mental activities involved in directed skill acquisition. Washington, DC: Storming Media; 1980. https://apps.dtic.mil/dtic/tr/fulltext/u2/a084551.pdf. Accessed 13 Jun 2020.

11. Whitehouse D. Renaissance genius: Galileo Galilei & his legacy to modern science. New York, NY: Sterling Publishing; 2009. p. 219. ISBN 978-1-4027-6977-1.

12. Cochrane A. One man's medicine. London: British Medic Journal (Memoir Club); 1989. p. 82.

13. Bryson B. The body. London: Penguin Random House Publishers; 2019.

14. Kuhn TS. The structure of scientific revolutions. New York, NY: New American Library; 1986.

15. Laudan L. Progress and its problems: towards a theory of scientific growth. Berkley, CA: University of California Press; 1977.

16. Merton RK. On the shoulders of giants. A shandean postscript. The post-Italianate edition. Chicago, IL: University of Chicago Press; 1993. p. XIV. ISBN 9780226520865.

17. Meleis A. Theoretical nursing: development and progress. New York, NY: J.B. Lippencott Company; 1985.

18. Hunt J. Indicators for nursing practice: the use of research findings. J Adv Nurs. 1981;6(3):189–94.

19. Carper BA. Fundamental patterns of knowing in nursing. Adv Nurs Sci. 1978;1(1):13–23.

20. Benner P, editor. From novice to expert. New York, NY: Addison Wesley; 1984.

21. McKenna HP. Critical care: does profusion of evidence lead to confusion in practice? Nurs Crit Care. 2010;15(6):285–90. PMID: 21040259.

22. Raulin, A. The Importance of Scientific Theory. Science. 1963;142:3590.

23. Bashford L, Slevin O, editors. Theory and practice of nursing: an integrated approach to caring practice. 2nd ed. Campion Press Ltd: Cheltenham; 2003. ISBN 0-7487-5838-0.

24. Toffler A. Future shock. New York, NY: Random House Publications; 1970.

Research Impact: An Analysis of Approaches in Health Sciences

8

In this business, it is all about making an impact

(Orton [1])

8.1 Introduction

In the 2014 REF, there were examples of health impact across all four Main Panels. In the Medical and Life Sciences Panel (Main Panel A), readers would not be surprised to learn that almost all the research impacts were health related. The exception is the expert panel for UoA6, which deals with agriculture and veterinary science. But even in this expert panel, human nutrition impacts were assessed. In the Physical Sciences and Engineering Panel (Main Panel B), the expert panels relating to computer science and engineering research assessed health impacts. Examples included, remote health monitoring, new designs of defibrillators, smart homes and computerised care planning.

In the Social Sciences Panel (Main Panel C), the expert panels of sports sciences, social work and social policy, business and management studies also assessed research impacts relating to health care. Examples included the contribution of sport and exercise to mental health, new policies relating to the care of older people and new models of healthcare administration. In the Arts and Humanities Panel (Main Panel D), the expert panels assessed the disciplines of music, drama and dance, art and design, and history reviewed research impacts pertaining to health. Examples included new therapies based on music and drama, new designs for health facilities and new histories of medicine.

> **Reflection Point 8.1 Health Impacts**
> Identify three research impacts relating to health care.
>
> There are endless examples of how health care can be impacted by research. Such impacts can take many forms. There follow some examples to illustrate the breadth of benefit:
>
> - Improved health or welfare outcomes.
> - Enhanced professional standards, ethics, guidelines or training.
> - Public health debate has been shaped or informed by research.
> - A new care or treatment product has been commercialised.
> - Changes in professional practice.
> - Public understanding, values, attitudes or behaviours towards health promotion has been changed.

H. P. McKenna, *Research Impact*, https://doi.org/10.1007/978-3-030-57028-6_8

- Changes to healthcare legislation, guidelines or regulations.
- More effective management of workplace practices.
- Improved quality, accessibility or efficiency of the health service.

Therefore, throughout the REF process, health impact has been generated by research across most of the 36 Units of Assessment. Some of these relate to economic impacts such as getting people back to work after illness or sales for a new healthcare technology. The impact can be social such as a reduction in depression due to social support or new community care initiatives for people with dementia. It could be cultural impact such as improving the well-being of disabled teenagers through music and art or increasing early cancer detection through exploring cultural values in multi-ethnic groups. It could also be technological impact such as increasing the connectivity of rural carers through the use of informational technology or enhancing independent living and lifestyle through smart home technology. Moreover, impacts relating to health may cross a wide spectrum of academic disciplines and formed a considerable number of the impact case studies submitted in the 2014 REF.

8.2 An Analysis of Health Science Impacts Submitted in the 2014 REF

In this section, I analyse the research impact case studies submitted in the 2014 REF that focused on health sciences. The Expert Panel I selected was Allied Health Professions, Dentistry, Nursing and Pharmacy. When the key words 'health professions' are inserted into the search bar of the Research Impact database, 310 impact case studies are identified [2]. I read each in detail, noting issues such as what the research impact was, if and how the research underpinning the impact was funded, what research designs were used, and in what countries did the impact occur. Figure 8.1 shows the type of research impact reported.

From Fig. 8.1, it will come as no surprise to readers that most of the impact case studies focus on health, followed by political and society. It is surprising that health sciences research appears to have less of an impact on technology, the economy, the environment and no impact on culture. Considering that health professionals often influence economic productivity through health promotion and disease prevention and treatment, the low impact on the economy is surprising. Therefore, more consideration must be given to how healthcare research can have economic, as

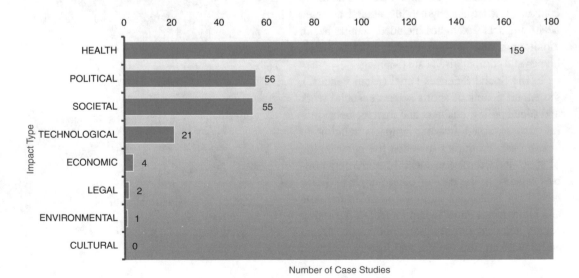

Fig. 8.1 Types of research impact reported in the 'Health Professions' case studies ($n = 310$)

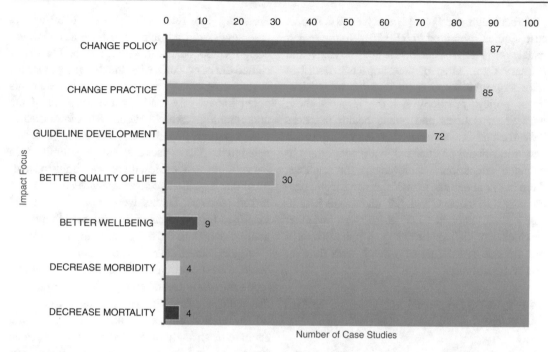

Fig. 8.2 Types of research impact pertaining to health sciences ($n = 310$)

well as health, impact. Otherwise, the UK Treasury may pose perceptive questions about why they should continue to fund such research.

Further in-depth analysis was undertaken on the research impacts pertaining to health (see Fig. 8.2).

From Fig. 8.2, the top three sources of research impact relate to changing policy, changing practice and the development of guidelines. Research impacts on improved quality of life come next and increased well-being and decreased morbidity and mortality have a much lower profile in these impact case studies. This is disappointing as it could be argued that well-being, morbidity and mortality are central to health care. Furthermore, an argument that I made earlier in this textbook is pertinent here. Simply influencing the development of guidelines, or changing policy and practice, is one step removed from real impact. In other words, just because research guidelines, policies and practises change does not always mean that people have benefited or will benefit.

As can be seen in Chap. 1, the REF definition of impact covers policy change. This can take many forms, all of which are legitimate within the definition and represent different stages of impact maturity. These include informing policy debate,

advising policy decisions, new policy legislation, policy implementation and improved public services as a result of new policy. But a complication is that it has been known for policies to sit on shelves. This may be because it was the policy of a previous government or administration. However, it might also be the case that nothing changed as a result of the policy, in fact things may have got worse.

The following example illustrates this point. In 2015 some colleagues and I undertook research into young male suicide in Northern Ireland [3, 4]. The resultant report fed into a new government policy on suicide prevention. However, in subsequent years, the rates of suicide did not decrease. The same argument can be made about clinical guidelines. Such guidelines can be introduced, but patient outcomes may not change for the better. This is important because 41% of case studies submitted to 'Clinical Medicine' in the 2014 REF were allocated to the topic 'Clinical guidance'. Furthermore, the history of health care is littered with examples of new practices such as workforce skill mix reviews, new model of care and treatment, etc. These initiatives undoubtedly changed practices, but it is uncertain if they really impacted on patient care.

Greenhalgh and Fahy [5] analysed 162 impact case studies submitted in REF 2014 to the expert panel for Public Health, Health Services and Primary Care. Most of the "impacts" described refer to implementation (of research into guidelines, policy, practice), not the impacts those guidelines, policies and public health practices have for end beneficiaries. If research informs a new educational practice but that practice fails to enhance educational achievement for students, there has not been any positive impact for end beneficiaries. In essence, Fig. 8.2. challenges healthcare researchers to ask themselves whether producing guidelines or changing policy has any real impact on the care of patients, their families and communities.

Reflection Point 8.2 Research Design and Impact

An interesting question to pose is whether different types of research design tend to drive research impact. Figure 8.3. shows the frequency of research designs underpinning these 310 impact case studies.

From Fig. 8.3, readers will note that 50 impact case studies did not appear to have any research design. Undoubtedly, they did, but the UoA concerned did not specify what the designs were. This is surprising considering that one of the elements of an impact case study is a description of the underpinning research. Figure 8.3 shows clearly that quantitative approaches to research predominated in the 310 impact case studies submitted. In some of the case studies, there was simply a statement that a qualitative approach was employed or mixed methods. Others were more explicit and identified focus groups or the Delphi technique or action research as the design used in the research.

Again, these results are not surprising. Randomised controlled trials, clinical trials and laboratory-based research are often referred to as the 'gold standard' in determining a cause and effect relationship (see Chap. 7). This would seem to be strongly linked to research causing an impact. One of the most surprising findings was the large part that systematic reviews generally and Cochrane systematic reviews specifically, had on creating research impact. Often the conclusion in most systematic reviews is a recommendation for more research to be undertaken.

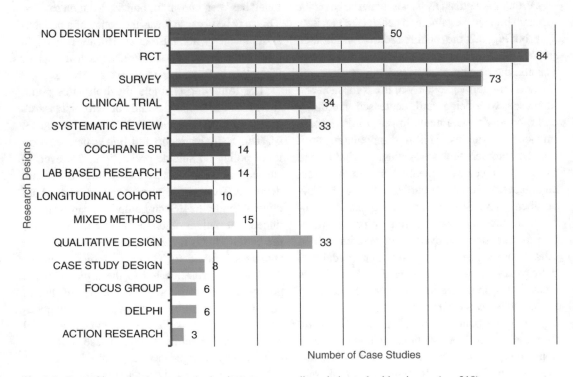

Fig. 8.3 Research approaches underpinning impact case studies relating to health sciences ($n = 310$)

A conclusion from Fig. 8.3. is that researchers need to ask themselves whether using qualitative research designs makes it harder for them to produce meaningful impact. Furthermore, why did action research, where researchers work with end users, scored so low? (See Chap. 6).

Research England [2] reported that all the impact case studies, that were non-redactable ($n = 6975$), had impact in every country in the world. This was a proud boast and showed the government and the treasury that the research undertaken in UK universities had global benefit. This encouraged the UK government to continue to invest public funds in university research. Figure 8.4. shows where in the world research pertaining to health sciences had impact.

Figure 8.4 indicates that UK health research that was submitted to this expert panel had most impact in the European Union. This may be due to the fact that many research studies were undertaken with colleagues from other European countries. One wonders if Brexit will have any effect on this pattern in future research assessment exercises. It can be seen that North America came second followed by Oceania. It is worth noting

that UK health research in this field has less impact in Africa and South America, probably two of the poorest continents represented in Fig. 8.4. These case studies tell a story of strong and diverse global impact. However, do UK taxpayers or charitable donors realise that their money funds research that benefits foreign multinationals, economies and governments rather than the UK, and if so, does this matter?

Further analysis was undertaken to see what the impact location was in the United Kingdom. Figure 8.5. shows that the largest number of UK impact case studies was in England, followed by Scotland and Wales and Northern Ireland. This may be related to the population sizes in these countries or the fact that England has a much larger number of universities than the other three UK countries. It may also be the result of there being more research funding in England compared to the other nations. However, Wales does have fewer universities than Scotland and yet the number of research impact case studies is the same.

It could be argued that high quality of research leading to outstanding research impact requires significant grant income. Figure 8.6 shows an

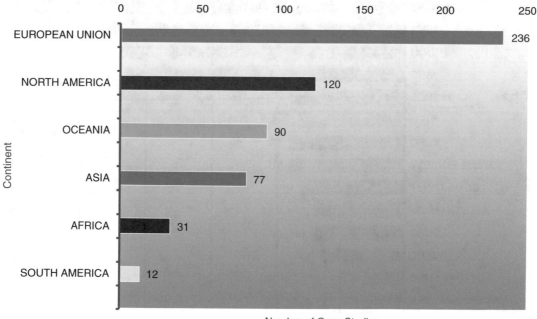

Fig. 8.4 Global location of the impact from health science research ($n = 310$)

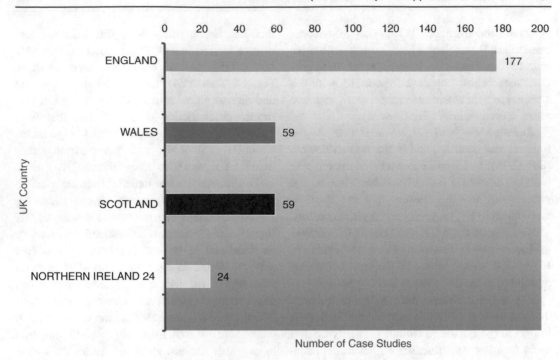

Fig. 8.5 UK location of the impact from health science research ($n = 310$)

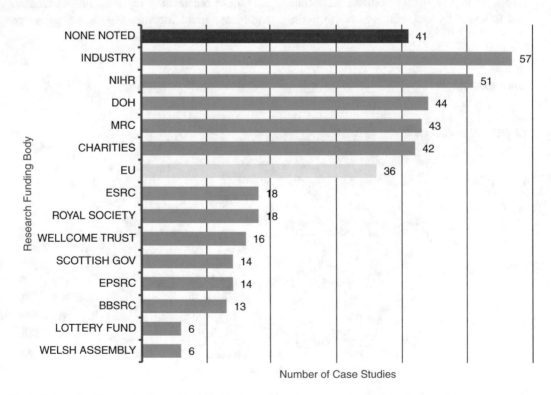

Fig. 8.6 Funding sources for the research impact ($n = 310$)

interesting set of trends. Perhaps the first thing to notice is that 41 of the impact case studies do not appear to have any research funding. If this is true, then one could claim that research impact is not contingent on having secured grant income. It may be that the underpinning research was funded, but this was not included in the case study. Furthermore, it is not possible to know how these 41 case studies were rated by the expert panel. They could have been rated as outstanding (4 star) or even unclassified; only panel experts will know how the case studies were rated, and this information is not available to universities. REF feedback only gives university leaders a rounded judgement of all three REF components—outputs, environment and impact.

The biggest funder of research in this field is industry. This might surprise readers but included here are pharmaceutical companies, medical device companies or organisations that have invested in research into the health and wellbeing of their staff. Of note is the fact that 36 of the case studies were funded by the European Union, probably through the Programme 8 or Horizon 2020 schemes. Once again, the effect of Brexit on funding from this source could have negative implications for future research impact. The UK National Institute of Health Research and the UK Department of Health are also big funders of health research. Health researchers do less well in winning research funding from the UK Research Councils (EPSRC, BBSRC, ESRC), or indeed the Wellcome Trust. It is unclear if health researchers do not apply for funding from these sources or, when they do, they are not successful. Included in the charity category are the Alzheimer's Society, British Heart Foundation, Cancer Research UK, etc. A lesson for health researcher from Fig. 8.6. is that they need to retain strong links with industry and apply for more Research Council funds.

8.3 A Comparison of Research Impact Quality with Other Components in REF

Expert panel assessors have to review outputs in both the output and impact components of REF. In Main Panel A (Health), these are mainly academic publications and for ease of understanding the term 'journal papers' will be used in this section. Therefore, journal papers can serve as evidence of a researcher's academic impact (submitted in the output component of REF) and as part of a case study showing evidence of impact (submitted in the impact component of REF).

Readers are reminded that all forms of output cited as underpinning research are considered on an equal basis by the expert panel assessors. In addition, the assessment of the journal papers used to underpin impact case studies will have no bearing on the quality assessment of those in the output component of REF. Furthermore, the journal papers may, but need not, have been submitted to a previous RAE or REF 2014.

There is a view from those who opposed the assessment of research impact that the pursuit of research impact within universities detracts from the quality of research conducted. In other words, the pressure in universities to generate research impact forces academics to conduct low-quality investigations of an applied nature. This challenge has been highlighted in Chap. 5.

Reflection Point 8.3 Research Quality and Impact Quality, the Relationship
Readers should consider whether high-quality research leads to high-quality impact.

Using REF 2024 data, I intend to investigate this perception by comparing each university's Grade Point Average (GPA) for research impact with its GPA for research outputs. I also want to compare each university's GPA for research impact with its GPA for overall quality (outputs, impact and environment). Whether the quality of research impact and the quality of research outputs are connected is an important question. In other words, does good research (represented as quality journal papers) have high impact, or does impact arise from superficial but 'flashy' research (represented as poorer quality journal papers)?

Before attempting this comparison, there is a caveat to consider. The impact case studies submitted had to be evidenced by journal papers linked to the underpinning research; these did not have to be same as those journal papers that were submitted in the output component within the same REF submission. So it is not possible to directly compare the quality of the journal papers that underpinned research impact with those journal papers that were submitted for assessment within the output component of the REF.

The reason for this merits rehearsing: Readers will remember that in each case study, UoAs could submit up to six journal papers as evidence of the impact quality (2 star or above; see Chap. 2). They did not all have to reach this standard, and for this reason, only some of them may have been reviewed. Remember also that UoAs could include a proxy (a prestigious award, grant or prize) for impact quality, and in this case, none of the six journal papers may have been reviewed. The implications for this is that only the rating for the impact is available for comparison not these underpinning journal papers.

This lack of consistency between the journal papers submitted as outputs and those submitted to underpin impact means that an intrinsic link with quality could only be established (or refuted) at a unit submission level. Using GPAs as comparisons, Terema et al. [6] found that there was a general trend towards high-quality work having high impact—the highest impact case studies (GPA = 4.0) compared well with the GPAs of 2.5–3.6 in the quality of research papers submitted as outputs. Similarly, the highest quality of papers submitted as outputs (GPA = 3.7) had very nearly the highest impact (GPA = 3.9).

Adams et al. [7] also found that journal papers included as both research outputs and, in case studies, showed relatively high impact both academically and societally. They postulated that there is every reason to expect that research that follows high academic standards (as evidenced by research papers) will also have societal value. This is not a new conclusion; as alluded to in Chap. 1, Vannevar Bush said much the same in his influential 1945 report for the United States government, Science, the Endless Frontier [8]. He argued that research which follows high academic standards can also be expected to have a broader societal value.

In their analysis of REF data, Terama et al. [6] also found a positive correlation between impact scores and the (overall research) quality scores. This intimates that impact is not being achieved at the expense of research excellence. Therefore, the positive correlation between research quality and research impact at institutional level suggested that there is little evidence that the pursuit of impact detracts from the quality of research. However, given selection bias within institutions, which meant that only high-quality research is submitted to the REF, this conclusion may not be surprising.

I decided to test this out with the 94 university submissions to the expert panel for dentistry, nursing, allied health professions and pharmacy in REF 2014. Readers will remember that the quality scores in the REF are between 0 star for unclassified and 4 star for the highest possible quality. Therefore, the lowest GPA that could be achieved was 0 and the highest was 4.0. For these 94 UoAs from submitting universities, the grade point average (GPA) for research impact was between 1.5 and 4.0 and the GPA for overall research quality was between 1.96 and 3.89. While the spread is different, there are similarities and a Pearson Product Moment Correlation test gave a 0.83 result. This represents a very close correlation between the quality of research impact and the overall quality (Outputs + Impact + Environment) for these 94 different units of assessment.

Figure 8.7 suggests that for these UoAs, the quality of research impact is highly correlated with the overall quality attained in the REF 2014. This supports the findings of Terama et al. [6], outlined above. Moreover, if the result had been that the impact had a high GPA and the overall research quality GPA was low, it could then be argued that impact was associated with low-

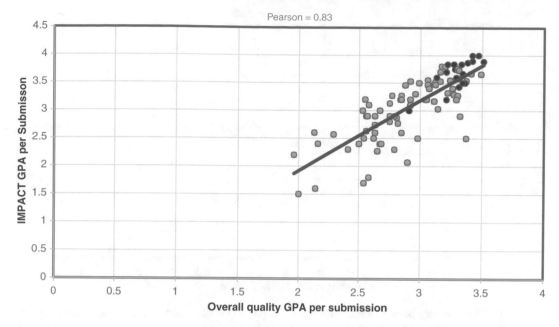

Fig. 8.7 Relationship between the overall quality and research impact in the REF 2014: (UoA3 $n = 94$). The red dots are research-intensive Russell group universities

quality research. Alternatively, if the impact had a low GPA and the overall quality GPA was high, it could be alleged that at a UoA, high-quality research was associated with low-quality impact. Neither of these was the case and those universities that score well in research impact also score well for quality research generally. In fact those Russell Group of research intensive universities, denoted by the red dots, tended to have high-quality impact and high overall quality.

But would this close positive relationship hold up if I only calculated the GPA for those journal papers submitted in the research output component of REF and the research impact GPA for the same 94 UoAs? Obviously in this computation, the impact GPA remained between 1.5 and 4.0. However, the GPA for research outputs had a narrower spread of 2.03 and 3.43. When the Pearson Product Moment Correlation was applied (see Fig. 8.8), the result was 0.58, a lower positive relationship between research outputs and research impact.

Therefore, for the 94 university UoAs that submitted to this expert panel in the 2014 REF, the GPA correlation between the quality of research impact and the quality of research out-

puts was weaker than that between the quality of research impact and the overall quality for those submissions. Nonetheless, it is accepted that at 0.58, there is still a positive relationship between the GPA for impact case studies and the GPA for outputs.

8.3.1   A Historical Exploration of Research Impact and Related Publications

I want to segue away from health for a moment to take a historical perspective on this link between research impact and academic outputs. There is a tradition where famous scientists achieved outstanding impact from their research, and yet they were not very prolific in terms of the number of publication produced and their citation indices [9]. Isaac Newton was famous for formulating the laws of gravitation, yet he produced only four publications giving him the H-Index of 4. Michael Faraday was known as the father of electricity, but the H-Index for his 23 publications was 18. Charles Darwin, the founder of evolution, had the H index of 27 for his 29 publications. Gregor

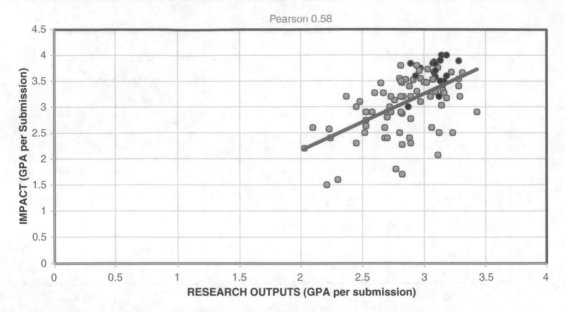

Fig. 8.8 UoA3 relationship between research outputs and impact in the REF 2014 (UoA3 $n = 94$). The red dots are research-intensive Russell group universities

Mendel's major contribution to genetics produced one publication, giving him the H-Index of 1. Max Planck discovered energy quanta, for which he won the Nobel prize. He produced 32 publications and has the H-Index of 27. Francis Crick helped discover the structural makeup of DNA and was jointly awarded the Nobel Prize. However, his 65 publications gained him the H-Index of 54.

No one could deny that the outstanding research impact was created by these researchers. Yet their publication metrics as measured by the H-Index are relatively modest. Perhaps that is because the quality of their publications are being judged by modern criteria. Nonetheless, the same outcome applies to a more recent Nobel laureate. In Chap. 5, I stated that Peter Higgs discovered the Higgs Boson and was honoured by the Nobel Committee. The Higgs Boson is impactful because it gives mass to the universe, people, buildings, planets, etc. In 2016, the Higgs Centre for Innovation, opened in Edinburgh and at the time Peter Higgs claimed that he would not get a job in it if he was judged on the number of publications and his H-Index. Higgs may also have the lowest H-index of any Nobel Prize winner. He has five publications, giving him an H-index of 5. These examples show that scientists who achieve outstanding research impact may have a modest amount of quality publications.

8.4   Impact Case Studies for REF2014 Relating to Health Care

In this section, I will describe and discuss four impact case studies (from hundreds) that were submitted in the REF 2014. These are from four different expert panels within Main Panel A representing UoA1, UoA2, UoA3 and UoA4. Each of these were rated as outstanding (4 star quality). I know this impact profiles for each of these university UoAs scored four star. For reason of space, I will present a short synopsis of each, hopefully providing readers with a flavour of outstanding impacts pertaining to health benefits. In case some readers want to follow up, I include the web link to the full case study. When reading these examples, readers might wish to refer to the guidelines on impact case studies in Chap. 2.

8.5   UoA1: Clinical Medicine—The University of Bristol

https://impact.ref.ac.uk/casestudies/CaseStudy.aspx?Id=40152

8.5.1   Title

Use of aspirin and high dietary fibre to prevent and reduce deaths from bowel and other cancers, influencing global policy on cancer prevention and major public health campaigns ('five-a-day').

8.5.2   Summary of the Impact

Clinical trials involving the Bristol group show that the incidence of bowel cancer has fallen in patients who take aspirin. Moreover, aspirin use after diagnosis of bowel cancer has reduced colorectal cancer mortality. Furthermore, a high fibre diet also lowers the risk of bowel cancer. These studies led to national public health initiatives (such as the 'five-a-day' campaign) that have been instrumental in increasing public awareness of the importance of aspirin and dietary fibre in reducing the risk of bowel cancer and in establishing international guidelines on dietary advice.

8.5.3   Underpinning Research

Bowel cancer is the second most common cause of cancer-related deaths in the UK, with 16,000 deaths a year. Worldwide, 600,000 such deaths occur annually. This research was been funded by five consecutive Cancer Research UK programme grants, running until 2015. Work undertaken between 1993 and 1995 at Bristol was the first to show that the candidate chemopreventive agent, butyrate (bacterial fermentation product of dietary fibre), and other short chain fatty acids, induced apoptosis (programmed cell death) in human colorectal adenoma and carcinoma cells. The findings that aspirin and COX-2 selective agents induced apoptosis led to the important hypothesis that these might also be used as adjuvants for bowel cancer as well as for cancer prevention.

8.5.4   References to the Research

Here the case study included six references to original research in journals such as the *Lancet and Cancer Research*. Grants of over £4m from

prestigious bodies were also highlighted in this section.

8.5.5   Details of the Impact

The case study described a number of impressive impacts from the underpinning research. These included: (1) impact of CRUK publications on committee invitations and development of clinical trials; (2) aspirin significantly reduces colorectal cancer incidence in HNPCC hereditary bowel cancer patients (CAPP2 trial) at very high risk of bowel cancer; (3) impact of high dietary fibre on reducing the risk of bowel cancer in the general population and increasing public awareness; (4) impact of aspirin as an adjuvant therapy for colorectal cancer; (5) impact of aspirin on saving lives in several major cancers, not just colorectal cancer; (6) impact of Bristol publications on national and international public awareness and public understanding of cancer prevention; (7) international impact of Bristol publications and clinical trials on public understanding and (8) impact of Bristol's Colon Cancer Group publications on clinical trials development.

8.5.6   Sources to Corroborate the Impact

The case study had 13 corroborative sources listed, from publications, to guidelines to media reports on the research and its impact.

8.5.7   Comment

This is an interesting impact case study. The title is descriptive but seems a little long. The summary shows that there are more than one impact, and each is described briefly. The underpinning research stated the research problem and that the Bristol team has been involved in a number of studies on how and why dietary fibre and aspirin prevent colon cancer. The reference section confirms for the assessor that the quality threshold of 2 star has been exceeded through the journals cited and the prestigious nature of the funding. Citations are included with each publication, and this will not be necessary in the next REF (see Chap. 2).

The description of the impact is well written and details seven different impacts from the underpinning research. By doing this, they risked diluting the reach and significance of all the impacts. The corroborating sources are extensive. From Chap. 2, readers will note that up to ten corroborative sources can be used in each impact case study, but there is some flexibility. However, because the case study is well constructed and the evidence is clear, these sources may not have been audited to confirm the impacts. The concepts reach and significance are not mentioned, leaving the assessors to find the evidence for these.

8.6   UoA2: Public Health, Health Services and Primary Care— The University of Oxford

https://impact.ref.ac.uk/casestudies/CaseStudy.aspx?Id=9537

8.6.1   Title

Statin therapy for preventing heart attacks and strokes.

8.6.2   Summary of the Impact

Changes in prescribing have strongly influenced the labelling of statin medication internationally, treatment guidelines, and the resulting changes in prescribing have contributed to reductions in mortality and morbidity from heart attack and ischaemic stroke in many countries. There is also a statement that there is clear evidence on the cost-effectiveness of statins.

8.6.3   Underpinning Research

This section outlined the research that has been ongoing since 1994 including investigations on 20,000 patients. It described further research in the form of clinical trials and meta-analyses. The results showed the positive effects from lowering cholesterol in patients with or without cardiovascular risk and in patients with kidney disease.

8.6.4   References to the Research

The six references from the underpinning research were all published in the *Lancet* with a brief description of the findings from each. There is also an outline of the prestigious funding sources.

8.6.5   Details of the Impact

This section describes succinctly the impact of a statin regimen on the reduction of the risk of heart attacks, strokes and revascularisation procedures in both high-risk and healthy people and people with kidney disease. This work has influenced treatment guidelines and statin medication labelling internationally. All the major national and international healthcare policy guidelines on cardiovascular disease prevention have been influenced by this work.

8.6.6   Sources to Corroborate the Impact

Ten corroborating sources are included, including website, NICE guidelines, testimonials, publications and media articles.

8.6.7   Comment

The title is concise and precise, and the summary clearly states the many important impacts associated with this submission. The underpinning research showed the long lead in time for the underpinning research and briefly described what each study found and how that formed the foundations for the next study. The six references illustrate the high quality of the publications. The short description accompanying each provides a proxy indicating that the 2 star quality threshold for the research was exceeded. Interestingly the cost-effectiveness is mentioned in the summary but not in the details of the impact. Media attention is included. Nonetheless, the impact of the research on three difference beneficiaries shows the reach and significance. The corroborating sources show breadth and depth of validation. Here too, the concepts reach and significance are not mentioned in the case study, leaving the assessors to find the evidence for these.

8.7 UoA3: Allied Health Professions, Dentistry, Nursing and Pharmacy—The University of Nottingham

https://impact.ref.ac.uk/casestudies/CaseStudy.aspx?Id=28016

8.7.1 Title

Delivering public health services through community pharmacy.

8.7.2 Summary of the Impact

The summary highlights a number of research impacts: has been used by the UK government in their drive to improve the nation's public health; informed the 2008 White Paper 'Pharmacy in England: Building on Strengths—Delivering the Future'; cost-effective delivery of public health services; an increase in public awareness and access to these services; and the Government is using the research to develop, implement and evaluate public health practice in pharmacy.

8.7.3 Underpinning Research

The research projects underpinning the claimed research impacts have been conducted over a number of years going back to the year 2000. At that time, the UK government established Health Action Zones. The teams carried out several evaluation studies of the health promotion initiatives ongoing within these HAZs. Systematic reviews were also undertaken and contributed to the impacts.

8.7.4 References to the Research

The references supplied include academic papers in good-quality journals and reports. These were published between 2001 and 2006. Grants were also listed from the Department of Health, local authorities and Boots the Chemist.

8.7.5 Details of the Impact

This section comprehensively described the impacts listed in the above summary. It shows how the research has informed government policy on the contribution that community pharmacists can make to public health. Having such services on the high street has engaged the public is many health promotion schemes, of which there were positive impacts. These include smoking cessation, emergency hormonal contraception, influenza immunisation, diabetes and drug misuse.

8.7.6 Sources to Corroborate the Impact

These sources cover nine different corroborations, and includes government policy and testimonial, reports of health strategies and a statement from Royal Society.

8.7.7 Comment

Pharmacists are developing from being dispensers of medications to having a key role in the promotion of health and the prevention of illness. The title encapsulates exactly the essence of the impact case study in a concise way and commences with an action verb. The summary expands this by listing a number of public health impacts that have resulted. The underpinning research projects are mainly evaluation studies and systematic reviews. It is of good quality and covers a period over a decade before the 2014 REF submission date. The references include literature reviews, original research papers and a report. They do however exceed the 2 star quality threshold. The funding is modest but appropriate for the type of research being undertaken. The public health impacts have changed government policy on community pharmacy showing that this workforce can have positive impacts on a range of health promoting behaviours. The nine corroboration sources are high-quality validators, but I noticed that several of them were linked to webpages, which, the REF guidelines show, assessors did not have to follow. Again, for this case study, the concepts reach and significance are not mentioned, leaving the assessors to find the evidence for these.

8.8 UoA4: Psychology, Psychiatry and Neuroscience—The University of Stirling

https://impact.ref.ac.uk/casestudies/CaseStudy.aspx?Id=44433

8.8.1 Title

Changing policy and practice in the prevention of suicide and self-harm.

8.8.2 Summary of the Impact

Here too both impacts are described succinctly—one influencing policy and the other influencing practice.

8.8.3 Underpinning Research

In this section, the research problems are clearly articulated in the first paragraph. The theoretical underpinning for the research is outlined in the third paragraph, and the research programme is addressed in the fourth paragraph.

8.8.4 References to the Research

The references are mostly academic papers in high-quality journals with a book chapter. The list of research grants is impressive.

8.8.5 Details of the Impact

This section outlines three distinct types of impact on (1) government policy, (2) development of clinical guidelines for the management of self-harm and suicide risk and (3) using theory to inform practice in terms of the identification and assessment of risk. Each is described in detail.

8.8.6 Sources to Corroborate the Impact

The corroborating sources include reports, debates, strategies and clinical guidelines.

8.8.7 Comment

The title is self-explanatory and hints at two different impacts. It also starts off with an action verb. The summary provides more detail of the two impacts claimed. The underpinning research section does not provide much information on the actual studies conducted or their methodologies. This reference section includes seven references, even though the upper limit is six, and, apart from one, they are all mainly led by O'Connor. This might suggest that the team is small, or this could be a one man show. They exceed the 2 star quality threshold. The research grants are from prestigious sources and are spread over time, and the amounts are substantial. The impact section identifies three impacts, which is one more than specified in the title or summary. The impact section shows that the research has influenced the development or policy, guidelines and practice nationally and internationally. This is impressive, but it would be much better if there were data on how this has prevented the number of suicides and self-harm episodes. There are 12 corroborating sources, even though 10 is the maximum required. But as highlighted above, there can be some flexibility. Once again, there was no explicit mention of reach or significance.

This is a really interesting impact case study. It stimulates interest in an assessor as to whether the policy was implemented and whether the practice actually reduced death by suicide or morbidity through self-harm. It will be interesting to see whether it is a continued one in the next REF, and if so, will there be data on actual lives saved. Suicide is a major public health issue and like most public health topics, it is almost impossible to state with certainty how many people were affected. For instance, using another example of a public health problem—Covid-19—it would be really difficult to quantify how many people did not contract the virus as a result of policy!

8.9   Summary

Health care is a global phenomenon, and so it is not surprising that many research impact case studies in the 2014 REF pertained to health benefits from underpinning research. This chapter starts by highlighting how impacts for most of the submitted units of assessment focused on health. There follows an analysis of 310 health-related impact case studies that were submitted in the REF. It showed the types of impacts, where the impact took place, what research designs were used and whether or not the underpinning research was funded. The next section reported on another study where I compared the quality of research publications with research impact and the overall quality of 94 individual UoAs. Finally,

four impact case studies from health-related expert panels were described. These were given the highest possible rating of 4 star (outstanding).

References

1. Orton R. 2020. https://www.wwe.com/superstars/randy-orton.
2. Research England. REF2014 research impact case study database; 2020. https://impact.ref.ac.uk/casestudies/.
3. Cutcliffe J, McKenna H, Keeney SR, Jordan J. 'Straight from the horse's mouth': rethinking and reconfiguring services in Northern Ireland in response to suicidal young men. J Psychiatr Mental Health Nurs. 2013;20:466–72. https://doi.org/10.1111/jpm.12012.
4. Jordan J, McKenna HP, Keeney SR, Cutcliffe JR, Stephenson C, Slater P, McGowan IW. Providing Meaningful Care: Learning. From the Experiences of Suicidal Young Men. Qualitative Health Research. 2012;X9X:1–13. https://doi.org/10.1177/1049732312450367.
5. Greenhalgh T, Fahy N. Research impact in the community-based health sciences: an analysis of 162 case studies from the 2014 UK Research Excellence Framework. BMC Med. 2015;13:232. https://doi.org/10.1186/s12916-015-0467-4.
6. Terema E, Smallman M, Lock SJ, Johnson C, Zaltz Austwick M. Beyond academia – interrogating research impact in the research excellence framework. PLoS One. 2016;11(12):e0168533.
7. Adams J, Bornmann L, Haunschild R. Excellence is useful. Research Professional 18 Apr 2019, 08:00; 2019. https://www.researchprofessional.com/0/rr/news/europe/views-ofeurope/2019/4/Excellence-isuseful.html?utm_medium=email&utm_source=rpMailing&utm_campaign=personalNewsDailyUpdate_2019-04-18#sthash.ceMccvrH.dpuf.
8. Bush V. Science: the endless frontier, a report to President Truman outlining his proposal for post-war U.S. science and technology policy. Washington, DC, USA: United States Government Printing Office; 1945.
9. Belikov AV, Belikov VV. A formula to estimate a researcher's impact by prioritizing highly cited publications. BioRxiv. 2016; https://doi.org/10.1101/058990.

Research Impact: A Global Perspective on Its Assessment

9

'You cannot get through a single day without having an impact on the world around you. What you do make a difference, and you have to decide what kind of difference you want to make'. Jane Goodall [1]

9.1   Introduction

Global higher education institutions need some mechanism of assessing the payback for the funding they receive for university research. The public is becoming increasingly vocal on how universities are charging their children's large tuition fees, yet they as taxpayers are also contributing millions to the research activities of the same universities. It comes as no surprise that across the globe universities are being held to account for how they use public funds. If it can be demonstrated that tax payers' investment in research leads to social, economic and cultural impact, some of the criticism can be assuaged. One of the countries that initially considered the assessment of research impact was Australia.

9.2   Australia

The first attempt globally to comprehensively capture the socio-economic impact of research across all disciplines was undertaken for the Australian Research Quality Framework (RQF), using a case study approach [2]. The RQF was developed to demonstrate and justify public expenditure on research, and as part of this framework, a pilot assessment was undertaken by the Australian Technology Network. Researchers were asked to evidence the economic, societal, environmental and cultural impact of their research within broad categories, which were then verified by an expert panel.

It concluded that case studies could provide enough qualitative and quantitative evidence for reviewers to assess the impact arising from research [3]. To evaluate impact, these case studies were interrogated and verifiable indicators assessed to determine whether research had led to reciprocal engagement, adoption of research findings or public value. Therefore the RQF pioneered the case study approach to assessing research impact; however, with a change in government in 2007, this framework was never implemented in Australia; rather, it found its way into the UK REF in 2014.

More recently, the Australian Government considered adopting the UK model of research assessment. Professor Margaret Sheil, the CEO of the Australian Research Council that led the country's first research assessment scheme, called it

'Excellence in Research for Australia' (ERA). As it developed, it became different and, in some ways, better than the UK exercise. For one, it ranked refereed academic journals, something the UK has always been reluctant to do, probably because of possible legal challenges from publishing houses or that quality articles can be found in all journals. The first ERA also included an assessment of the impact of research—something that, at that time, was missing from the UK exercise. However, the Australian Minister for Innovation, Industry and Research, The Hon Kim Carr dispensed with the impact assessment as it was seen as too problematic to develop a metric that would be accepted as valid and acceptable across a number of academic disciplines.

The UK adoption of research impact assessment in the 2014 REF caused a rethink in Australia. In 2018, officials in the Australian Research Council (ARC), in charge of implementing ERA, revisited research impact. Australian universities were required to prove that their research provides concrete benefits for the taxpayers and the government who fund it. The ARC introduced an Engagement and Impact Assessment approach to run alongside the ERA exercise. This followed a 2017 pilot of the Engagement and Impact Assessment.

The ARC has defined engagement as: *the interaction between researchers and research end-users outside of academia, for the mutually beneficial transfer of knowledge, technologies, methods or resources* [4]. This metric allows universities to demonstrate and be rewarded for engaging industry, government and others in research, even if it does not directly or immediately lead to impact.

Engagement is assessed on four key metrics and an engagement narrative. These metrics are focused on funding provided by research users such as businesses or individuals outside the world of academia who directly use or benefit from the research conducted by university-based academics. The four metrics are cash support, sponsored grants from end-users, research commercialisation income and how much income is made per researcher. As can be seen from these four metrics, the initial focus was on commercial engagement. As stated in Chap. 4, the UK government assesses and rewards

such engagement in the Knowledge Exchange Framework [5]. While it is also organised through the UK Research and Innovation Office, the KEF is a separate initiative to REF.

In ERA the definition of impact was amended to include 'culture', which was not part of the definition applied in the pilot exercise. This amendment arose from concerns raised by the academic community around quantifying and qualifying impacts that vary significantly across different academic fields. They had raised questions such as how does one compare an exhibition of art with the discovery of new biomarkers?

Impact has now been defined as: *the contribution that research makes to the economy, society and environment and culture beyond the contribution to academic research.* In essence, Australian researchers need to show the demonstrable contribution that research makes to the economy, society, culture, national security, public policy or services, health, the environment or quality of life, beyond contributions to academia.

Qualitative narratives about engagement are encouraged because they allow researchers to describe the important impacts they are achieving that quantitative metrics cannot easily capture. The case studies have to include the impact achieved, the beneficiaries and timeframe of the research impact and countries where the impact has occurred. They also comprise what strategies were employed to enable translation of research into real-world benefits. In the UK, this aspect is dealt with in the research environment component of the REF. The ERA evaluation criteria used by a panel of experts for each field of research provide gradings of '*high, medium* and *low*'. These criteria were much more welcome to universities than the benchmarks '*limited, emerging* and *mature*' used in the Australian pilot exercise.

The traditional research assessment metrics of grants, publication and citations are still included in the ERA. But unlike the UK, there is no money attached to the results. However, this may change as the assessment of impact becomes embedded in the review of university research. Because of the current lack of funding following quality ratings, there are concerns about complacency. Could it be that once the deadline has passed and the ERA submissions are done, everyone will simply return to what they perceive as normal academic business, until the next ERA? But as time progresses, there is a realisation that research impact and engagement assessment is going to be a permanent fixture in Australia.

In 2019, there was criticism of ERA from academic leaders in the arts, social sciences and humanities (ASH). This centred upon a divergence in quality assessment between these subjects and the science, technology, engineering and mathematics (STEM) disciplines, which is not seen in the UK REF. In the 2018 ERA, 80% of research in STEM was above the world average, up from 43% in the 2012 ERA. In contrast, 35% of research in ASH was above the world average, up just 8% since 2012. Could it be that the quality of research in ASH disciplines was not only poorer than the quality in science subjects, but that it was poorer than ASH research in the UK? One explanation is that ERA uses citation-based metrics for STEM evaluation and peer review for ASH, whereas in the REF, peer review is used across all disciplines. Because of this apparent anomaly, the Australian Research Council vowed to review ERA, although they did not admit that there was a problem.

Reflection Point 9.1 Mechanisms That Encourage Impact Through Engagement
From previous chapters, readers will be aware of the importance of researchers engaging with external research users for impact to be generated. Rehearse the best ways of doing this here and then compare that with the following five elements from Australia.

In *From Evidence to Impact*, [6] identified lessons from an evaluation of the Australian Development Research Award Scheme. They identified five elements worthy of note when considering research impact.

1. *Foundational facilitators: familiarity and prior engagement with research context and users.*
   They found that an understanding of the research context and of the relationships and networks between researchers and key end users or influencers was foundational to

impact. This included an understanding of the local political, policy and socio-cultural context. Knowledge of local context prior to planning the research, and mechanisms to stay abreast of changes, were key facilitators for the generation of impact. In particular, three mechanisms were found to contribute: (a) inclusion of external in-country partners in research teams; (b) appointment of an advisory committee of key stakeholders and (c) previous or formative work in the setting. Long-established relationships of trust were key, particularly when the relationships were between end users and senior researchers, built up over a period. Continuity in the people who held research team positions and continuity in the positions held by key end users were also important in ensuring that interpersonal linkages helped drive impact.

2. *Planning for impact: intentional focus on impact and integrated methods for its achievement*
   Planning for impact or 'starting with the end in mind' was found to be key. Research that addressed a clear question or debate was more likely to be taken up and used in policy and practice than exploratory research that was designed to fill a gap in knowledge. Furthermore, projects with clearly targeted end users were twice as likely to influence policy and practice outcomes as projects with more broadly defined end users. In addition, teams that bridged sector silos and that had substantive roles for external partners and greater inclusion of target end users were more likely to influence policy and practice impacts.

3. *Engaging end users: proactive engagement and co-production of knowledge*
   Failure is associated with end user engagement occurring only at the beginning and end of the research process. Impactful research is synonymous with ongoing exchanges with end users in ways that aligned with their incentives, motivations and processes. Research findings were more likely to be used if they were *co-produced*, and if the timing of the results aligned with decision-making deadlines. The ability of external stakeholders to provide linkages with key individuals who

could assist with getting the research used and who supported take-up into their own policy or processes was crucial.

4. *Influential outputs: tailored, fit-for-purpose design of outputs*

   Because policymakers or members of national or regional bodies were unlikely to read long, dense reports, short outputs on aspects of the research most relevant to particular end user needs were found to facilitate research uptake. Easily digestible summaries were more likely to get stakeholders' attention than bulky tomes. This was further facilitated by short targeted guidelines or tools that contained clear practical recommendations and implementable actions.

5. Lasting engagement: ongoing engagement and continuity of relationships

   Long-term engagement between researchers and end users beyond the time-frames of the grant itself was particularly important in promoting the contribution to impact. Monitoring and evaluation of uptake and implementation of the research strongly improved outcomes and up-take. Moreover, it was important to be aware of the constraints to long-term engagement. These include time, funding and capacity restrictions for all partners (human resources, skills, priorities, etc.), as well as a lack of continuity in key positions in end user groups.

9.3   Hong Kong

Hong Kong has always followed the UK's approach to research assessment. The University Grants Committee had five such exercises in 1993, 1996, 1999, 2006 and 2014. However, in terms of assessment structures and processes, it tends to be one exercise behind the UK. So, when the UK was undertaking REF in 2014, Hong Kong was still using the rules of the UK's previous 2008 model, the Research Assessment Exercise (RAE), which did not include the assessment of research impact. More recently, the University Grants Committee in Hong Kong has caught up with its latest RAE model, which was conducted in 2020. This has been the first time

that Hong Kong RAE has included research impact as part of its review of research quality. This was done in an attempt to encourage the conduct of research of broader relevance with high economic and social benefits. However, the first page of the Hong Kong RAE 2020 guidelines directs readers to the equivalent document for the 2014 REF. This is surprising considering that it could refer them to the REF2021 guidelines.

Therefore, their approach is very much based on the UK 2014 REF with reach and significance being the criteria for assessment, and these are applied to submitted case studies from Hong Kong universities. Furthermore, the universities had to show how they encouraged impact, an aspect the UK REF has included within its research environment component.

The Hong Kong definition of research impact also has similarities with the UK REF. These are to ensure demonstrable contributions, beneficial effects, valuable changes or advantages that research qualitatively brings to the economy, society, culture, public policy or services, health, the environment or quality of life, whether locally, regionally or internationally and that are beyond academia.

For Hong Kong universities, research impact includes the reduction or prevention of harm, risk, cost or other negative effects and impacts on teaching or students that extend significantly beyond the submitting university, or on other fields. As with REF 2014, it excludes impacts to academic advances and impacts on students, teaching or other activities within the submitting university. Considering that for the next REF, the UK has changed its rules to include impact on teaching and learning within the submitting university, it seems that Hong Kong is still one assessment model behind the UK.

Reflection Point 9.2 The Influence of the UK in Hong Kong's RAE

It can be seen above that there is a major UK influence in how Hong Kong reviews its research quality. Try and identify some advantages and disadvantages with this.

O'Sullivan [7] criticises Hong Kong's approach to research assessment as a throwback to colonialism. He points out that there are UK assessors on all of the assessment panels and that UK consultants have been employed to assist Hong Kong universities in their RAE preparations. He asked how would the UK academy feel if Hong Kong assessors were reviewing UK research. Another issue that bears consideration is whether the increasing Beijing influence on Hong Kong society generally, and universities particularly, will see an end to their RAE.

The 2019 riots in Hong Kong and the influence of the Covid-19 virus have damaged its reputation as a global financial centre. Therefore, the focus on research impact for the betterment of society, culture and the economy is appropriate. Furthermore, the UK has one of the most advanced systems of assessing quality internationally and by adopting it, Hong Kong did not have to create its own system. In addition, as can be seen above, many countries have learned from the REF experience and embraced aspect of it for their own approach; Hong Kong is not unique in doing this.

9.4 Canada

In recent years, there has been a 'big push' in Canada for researchers to demonstrate how they are contributing to solving the challenges faced by Canadians. Learned bodies such as the Federation for the Humanities and Social Sciences are contributing to the Canadian conversation about impact assessment. In 2009, the Canadian Academy of Health Sciences [8] produced a report entitled 'Making an impact: a preferred framework and indicators to measure returns on investment in health research'. It had five impact categories: advancing knowledge; capacity building; informing policies and product development; health and health sector benefits; and economic and social benefits.

The first two impact categories relate to academic benefit from publications, numbers of staff and research funding. To a large extent, these were focused on internal structures and processes. The other three impact categories concentrate on benefits outside the institution, and in accepted parlance, they would be broadly associated with societal impact. These are described in the following paragraphs.

The *Informing Policies and Product Development* category is self-explanatory. The types of indicators come across as a mixture of dissemination and impact:

- Healthcare guidelines and policy documents citations, e.g. regional plans, educational material, panel representatives
- Research references used as background for successful consulting and support activities
- Industrial patents and industrial collaborations
- Public information packages and dissemination activities
- Media exposure on radio, TV and social media

The advantage of these types of impact is that they can inform policy decision-making and the cost of generating such impact is nominal. The disadvantage is that there may be a time lag between the research being completed and the impact occurring. Because of the qualitative nature of some of the indicators, it can also be quite subjective.

The *Health and Health Sector Benefits* category includes more quantitative indicators compared to the previous impact category:

- Health data relating to incidence, prevalence, and mortality and quality-assisted life years (QALYs)
- Health determinants such as risk factors, educational and social level of cohesion, and pollution
- System changes including patient satisfaction, waiting lists, compliance and adherence to clinical guidelines, hospitalisation, length of inpatient stay, adverse effects/complications

The advantage of these types of impact is that they are robust and have relevance. As with the previous impact category, one of the disadvantages is the time lag between the research completion and the impact, but this problem is not unique to Canada. There are other disadvantages such as the feasibility of the impact and the cost of data collection, the latter being a particular burden for university researchers.

The final impact category is *Economic and Social Benefits* and here too the title is self-explanatory. As with the previous category, the indicators are mainly quantitative and include:

- Economic data such as rent, salaries, employments
- Licensing returns
- Product sales revenues
- Spin-out companies
- Health benefit such as QALY per healthcare dollar
- Well-being, happiness and level of social isolation
- Social benefits and socio-economic status

The advantage of these types of impact is that they are robust and have relevance. Here too the disadvantages include the feasibility and cost of data collection and the time lag between the research and the achievement of impact. However, there are other notable disadvantages including the possible underestimation of real impact and the difficulty in attributing the impact to the underpinning research because of confounding variables.

In 2007, Research Impact Canada (RIC) was established as a pan-Canadian network of universities committed to maximizing the impact of academic research for the public good in local and global communities [9]. It was established by York University and the University of Victoria, but others have joined since its foundation. It is committed to maximising the impact of academic research for the social, economic, environmental and health benefits of Canadians. What is unique about RIC is that, when measuring the impact of research, it also considers the traditional citation metrics alongside collaboration, mentoring and dialogue. Their approach blends both quantitative and qualitative methods of assessing impact to create a fuller picture of the true impacts of research.

As with other global assessment systems, the RIC uses a series of impact case studies to publicise the benefits accruing from research [9]. The following is a small sample of case studies including the Prairie Climate Centre, illustrating impact underpinned by research from the University of Winnipeg. It represents an outstanding example of making climate change meaningful for the general public. Another is the Reshaping Resilience Practices: A Co-Production Approach, where research was co-produced with vulnerable children and adults and those who support them. It informed a whole-system approach in schools and across local areas. Another impact case study was entitled A Driving Need: Study Connects Victoria Seniors with Volunteer Drivers. It focused on providing viable options for transportation of older people who are no longer able to drive. The social impact of these case studies (and many others) is obvious.

9.5   The United States of America

This trend towards generating and assessing research impact is also taking place in the United States. In particular, pressure has been building on researchers whose projects are funded with US aid money. Policymakers began asking questions such as what exactly are researchers doing for the US, its farmers and its people and how is that funding helping the US to be better? This is linked politically to the Trump administration's 'Make America Great Again' philosophy, incorporating the creation of wealth and economic growth.

One of the early initiatives that drove the research impact agenda in the USA was 'Star Metrics'. It was created in 2009 in direct response to requests from the White House Office of Management and Budget (OMB) and the Office of Science and Technology Policy (OSTP). They mandated that Federal agencies develop impact goals for their science and technology research [10]. It was also in direct response to the fervent desire to provide American federal taxpayers with precise information on the value of their investments in research. As with the REF and other research assessment systems around the world, it was widely believed that investments in science and research stimulate economic growth; the White House wanted to see the evidence.

The emergence of Star Metrics was influenced by the necessity on the part of the US federal government to gauge what impact national institutes of research were having on society generally and the economy in particular. The aim was to create a repository of data and tools that could be useful to assess the impact of federal research and development funding. The National Institutes of Health (NIH) and the National Science Foundation (NSF), under the auspices of the Office of Science and Technology Policy (OSTP), led this initiative with funding provided by the NIH, NSF, the U.S. Department of Agriculture, and the Environmental Protection Agency.

The federal administration was specifically interested in the impact of science funding with respect to job creation and economic expansion. It was accepted that this important question could not be creditably answered unless accurate data were collected and analysed. This was the catalyst for Star Metrics; before its advent, there were no mechanisms for linking science funding with impact or to engage the public meaningfully in discussions about scientific funding.

The goal of Star Metrics was to use existing administrative data from federal agencies and match them with existing research databases on economic, scientific and social outcomes. This was a straightforward task; Federal agencies already collected data on research funding at the individual researcher and institutional levels for the purposes of monitoring and managing grant awards. There was also a wealth of data existing on scientific and innovation outcomes such as citations, patents, business start-ups and intellectual property. In addition, there were existing tools to convey complex information about research to a lay audience. These sources of rich data formed the initial basis for the Star Metrics approach to gauging the impact of research funding and the disseminating of research findings through public engagement.

9.6   The European Union

The USA transferred some of the learning from the Star Metrics to Europe. In June 2011, participants from the European Commission, the USA and Japan met in Bellagio, Italy, at the Rockefeller Foundation Bellagio Centre and issued the Bellagio Statement. Its full and proper title was the *EU/US Roadmap to Measuring the Results of Investments in Science: The Bellagio Statement* [11].

As in the USA, there had been growth in European public and private investments in science and technology research. The results had been impressive and contributed to a range of innovations. These included the telecommunications and internet revolutions; providing better access to food, water and shelter; improving health care; combating environmental degradation and climate change; and helping to inform policies to promote social and economic security.

As can be seen throughout this textbook, it is a common objective for research assessments that they demonstrate that the tax payer is getting value for all the money invested in publicly funded research. This includes the social value of such funding, and national governments across the EU wanted transparency and accountability for research spending, and this had to be informed by the best possible data. It was necessary to reduce the reporting burden on researchers and a means of doing this was to exploit the enormous analytical power generated by advances in information technology. At the time of the Bellagio Statement's launch, Europe had still not emerged from the 2008 financial recession, meaning that there was enormous pressure on public funding. Therefore, more than ever before, the research community had to explain and justify its spending and show payback. There was also a great deal of scepticism across different European countries about both the marginal value of research spending and the chosen investment targets.

Despite the major strides already made in the USA through the interagency States-wide Star Metrics program, the need to have a shared approach with other EU nations was to be a challenge, hence the Bellagio conference. All participants agreed that research is a global activity with academics collaborating across borders. This led to an acceptance that the impact of research knows no frontiers and the need to form a mutually beneficial multi-national collaboration to document the impacts of investments in science. It established the foundations for a commitment to work together to develop a common framework to support the analysis of the impact of research funding.

The Bellagio Statement's focus on research impact had the desired ripple effect. It resulted in many European countries developing systems for the regular review of university research excellence. Sivertsen [12] helpfully divided the systems used into four categories:

- The purpose of funding allocation is combined with the purpose of research evaluation. The evaluation is organised at intervals of several years and based on expert panels applying peer review. Bibliometrics may be used to inform the panels. Examples of countries in this category are Italy, Lithuania, Portugal and the United Kingdom.
- The funding allocation is based on a set of indicators that represent research activities. Bibliometrics is part of the set of indicators. The indicators are used annually and directly in the funding formula. Examples of countries in this category are Croatia, the Czech Republic, Poland and Sweden.
- Similar to the previous category, but the set of indicators represents several aspects of the universities' main aims and activities, not only research. Bibliometrics are employed as part of the set of indicators. Examples of countries in this category are Flanders (Belgium), Denmark, Estonia, Finland, Norway and Slovakia.
- As in the previous category, but bibliometrics is not part of the set of indicators. Examples of countries in this category are Austria and the Netherlands.

The UK was the first European country to include research impact in a national evaluation of research quality linked to university funding.

However, since Sivertsen wrote his paper, many others are now showing a keen interest in including the review of research impact in their national exercises. In October 2017, a meeting of European senior policymakers in Estonia called for the EU's definition of research impact to be broadened. Delegates took the view that simply analysing research impact in terms of article citations was disastrous [13].

Speakers at the event called for a rejuvenated understanding of impact that includes the value of research for society. There was a call for better public engagement on impact. They stressed their desire to show the public that research funders and university investigators need to understand the problems that the public think are important. At the meeting, the EU Commissioner of Research, Science and Innovation, Carlos Moedas asserted that he wanted impact to be a major priority in the following European Framework Programme [13]. Since then, the assessment of research impact has taken a more important role in Europe.

The European Commission has tasked a consortium with analysing the impact of researchers funded through Framework 7, the EU's 2007–2013 R&D programme. The aim of the project was to complement the reports by identifying outputs such as intellectual property rights, outcomes such as companies created, and impacts such as improvements in people's quality of life. This set the impact agenda for all future EU funding schemes.

After the 2017 Estonian conference, a public consultation was launched on the impact of research and innovation in Europe. The consultation called on researchers, funders and policymakers to put forward proposals on how to get more impact from European research and innovation. One of the questions included in the consultation sought views on what European advances in science and technology had the biggest impact. Options for this question included the discoveries of the structure of DNA and the risks of climate change, as well as the invention of Skype, an Estonian internet services company. This illustrated that research funded and conducted in Europe had global reach and significance.

Also in 2017, the League of European Research Universities (LERU) widened its membership. Its sole purpose is to influence policy in Europe and to develop best practice through mutual exchange of experiences. LERU makes high-level policy statements, provides analyses and makes recommendations for policymakers, universities, researchers and other stakeholders [14]. It asserted that universities should embrace efforts by policymakers to make them demonstrate societal impact. It outlined that the research impact agenda is fully compatible with universities' historical fundamental missions of knowledge creation and transmission and should be fully embraced. It stated that this should go hand-in-hand with increased engagement with governments, funders, industry, civil society and members of the public to develop a better understanding of research impact.

There follows a small sample of the many European countries that have included research impact in their assessment of research quality.

9.6.1   Sweden

The Swedish Research Council is an agency under the authority of the Ministry of Education and Research, responsible for funding and developing basic research in all academic disciplines. It has a leading role in developing Swedish research to the highest scientific quality, thereby bringing benefit to Swedish society.

In 2014, the Swedish Research Council was tasked by the Swedish Government to evaluate the quality of the clinical health research conducted across the seven County Councils. These cover all of Sweden and are funded for research by the Swedish taxpayers. Each County Council has a nearby university and a university hospital, and jointly all three are referred to as an ALF region. ALF is shorthand for the agreement between national government and the seven regions that addresses medical education and training, clinical research and the development of health and medical care.

The ALF agreement was renewed on 1 January 2015, and one of the new inclusions was a novel quality-based funding allocation model. From 2019, the distribution of 20% of the ALF funding was to be based on the results of an evaluation of the quality of clinical research. This research assessment exercise was also referred to as the 'ALF'. It was decided that this was to be conducted using three independent panels to evaluate:

- The scientific quality (ALF Panel 1)
- The clinical significance and societal impact of the clinical research (ALF Panel 2)
- The prerequisites of the clinical research (ALF Panel 3)

Therefore, in 2019, research impact was going to be included for the first time as a criterion for the allocation of public funds for research in Sweden (albeit only 20% for this first exercise). As in the UK REF, there was much consternation from the Swedish universities who were concerned that this new approach might disadvantage them. Senior members of the Swedish Research Council visited the REF Team in London to discuss how best to approach this assessment. The Swedish Research Council appointed Professor Hugh McKenna to chair one of the panels, as he had chaired an expert panel in the 2014 REF.

It can be seen above that the ALF Panel 2 clearly assesses research impact. However, one of the roles of the ALF Panel 1 was to assess the clinical relevance of publications. All the assessors in ALF Panel 1 were from outside Sweden, mainly from the other Scandinavian countries and other European countries. The assessors had to consider the importance of each publication in relation to the potential impacts of research in that area. Three questions were posed:

- How significant is the contribution of this publication to the knowledge base in the area into which it may be classified?
- Which are the potential impacts from research in this area?
- What is the reach and significance of these potential impacts?

The REF definitions of reach and significance were employed. ALF Panel 2 assessed societal impact, which was impact arising in locations other than clinical practice. This included, the economy, society, public policy and services, production and environment. ALF Panel 2 also assessed clinical significance, which included impacts on patient care and health that arise in clinical practice. Clinical significance encompasses, for instance, new treatments or diagnoses of a particular disease, guidelines for treatment, or phasing out redundant methods (disinvestment).

So there are several similarities between the ALF and the REF. One relates to research impact beyond academia assessed as reach and significance. Another relates to the underpinning research. This is the extent to which the research conducted in each ALF region was considered to have made a substantial and distinct contribution to the impact claimed. Another similarity includes the extent to which the processes and strategies of the ALF region may be considered to have contributed to the impact in the described context. In the UK, this is included in the Research Environment component of the REF.

Across all the ALF Panels, there were three quality ratings that could be allocated by the assessors. These were:

- *Very high quality*, for those submissions that performed better than what is to be expected based on the amount of the allocated ALF funding.
- *Good–high quality* for those submissions indicating a performance at a level that is to be expected based on the amount of the allocated ALF funding.
- *Inferior quality* for those submissions indicating an inferior performance based on the amount of the allocated ALF funding, and/or in the unlikely event that the County Council failed to fully contribute to the evaluation.

Any submission that ended up in the inferior category will not be included in the ALF funding allocation. The Good–High submission received its normal allocation and those in the Very High Quality category received an increase in their normal funding allocation.

The ALF was well received and perceived as a success, particularly since no submission received an *Inferior Quality* rating. However, a different political party came into power in 2019, and the ALF was mothballed after the first exercise. Nonetheless, at the time of going to press, discussions are ongoing in the Swedish Research Council on how best to assess societal impact. One approach being considered is to place greater responsibility on universities to self-assess their contribution to research impact. This would be a similar approach to Research Impact Canada.

9.6.2   Holland

At around the same time that the Bellagio Statement was being developed in 2017, a framework called SIAMPI was evolving in the Netherlands. The acronym means **S**ocial **I**mpact **A**ssessment **M**ethods for research and funding instruments through the study of **P**roductive **I**nteractions between science and society. It was developed from the Dutch project, Evaluating Research in Context, and had a central theme of capturing 'productive interactions' between researchers and external stakeholders by analysing the networks that evolve during research programmes. Its evolution is founded on the accurate belief that interactions between researchers and external stakeholders are an important pre-requisite to achieving impact [10].

The SIAMPI project had three objectives:

- Identification of productive interactions between researchers and society in four research fields: nanotechnology, health, ICT and social sciences and humanities.
- Improvement of our understanding of the necessity of productive interactions as a condition for research to have a social impact.
- Development of approaches and tools for the evaluation of social impacts that are applicable in a range of fields and evaluation contexts, with a strong emphasis on the feasibility and sustainability of the suggested mechanisms.

Rather than a REF-based system to allocate public funding for research, the SIAMPI was intended to be used as a learning tool to develop a better understanding of how research interactions lead to social impact. The SIAMPI enhances the knowledge of the interactions between science and society and suggested innovative mechanisms to assess the social impact of research. It focused on three types of 'productive interactions' in creating social impacts: direct, indirect and financial interactions. It has been applied in healthcare, information and communications technology, nano-sciences and social sciences. It has also been used as a framework to map impactful interactions between researchers and society in France and Spain.

Case studies are used in the SIAMPI to reflect different fields of research and in different countries [15]. As in the UK REF, they present an acceptable approach to the assessment of the social impact of scientific research. They are written as a combination of qualitative narratives with quantitative indicators. In this way the results of impact assessments can be linked more easily to research activities and connected to policy, industry and the broader society.

While it was not a research assessment system in its own right, the SIAMPI set the foundations for what could be termed the Dutch REF—the Standard Evaluation Protocol (S.E.P.). This describes the methods used to assess research conducted at Dutch universities, the Royal Dutch Academy of Sciences and the Netherlands Organisation for Scientific Research (NWO). The evaluations are managed by QANU, a quality assurance agency. Every 6 years, these Dutch institutions have their research quality evaluated in the S.E.P.

Traditionally, as in most other countries, the S.E.P. approach has focused upon journal impact factors and citation indices. From 2021, this will change fundamentally. As in other countries, open science and an urgent need to tackle complex social and economic issues through collaboration are changing the perception and value of research metrics. The plan is that a review of social impact is to take precedence over the assessment of outputs and citations. Therefore, going forward, universities and research funders in the Netherlands have committed to judge sci-

entists on educational and social impact. At the time of going to press, this broader focus on societal impact is being enhanced, and Dutch research policymakers are seeking to learn from the next UK REF. This is more in line with the contemporary objectives of Dutch research and education institutions and what society requires of them.

9.7 Italy

In Italy there is a Three-Year Research Assessment Exercise (VTR). VTR is the formalised evaluation exercise launched by the Italian Government at the beginning of 2004, aimed to assess the research performance of academic institutions (universities and public research agencies) across scientific fields. The assessment relies heavily on peer review. Twenty panels, in charge of peer-reviewing, comprise 151 peers. Most of the peers come from Italian universities but a significant number come from abroad. Representatives from Italian public research agencies and from industry are also included. The VTR was mostly concerned with the assessment of academic impact rather than social impact. Therefore, and unsurprisingly, peer review of outputs formed the basis for the exercise [16].

More recently, regular research evaluation in Italy has become a decisive factor when it comes to justifying public investment decisions. It plays a central role in the transparent assessment of the social benefits and economic impacts achieved by research. The following bodies currently assess the quality of research in Italy and increasingly the assessment of research impact is gaining traction in at least two of these.

- The National Committee of Guarantors for Research (*Comitato Nazionale dei Garanti per la Ricerca—CNGR*)
- The National Agency for the Evaluation of the University and Research Systems (*Agenzia Nazionale di Valutazione del sistema Universitario e della Ricerca—ANVUR*)
- REPRISE, Register of Expert Peer-Reviewers for Italian Scientific Evaluation

9.7.1 National Committee of Guarantors for Research

The CNGR is a consultative body to the Ministry of Education, University and Research (MIUR). The committee is composed of seven high profile researchers, from Italy and abroad, and belonging to a wide range of disciplines.

9.7.2 National Agency for the Evaluation of the University and Research Systems

As a requirement under European policy, in 2010, Italy created the ANVUR (ANVUR), a public body which works to ensure the quality of higher education and research in Italy. Among the activities of ANVUR, it evaluates the quality of the processes, outcomes and products of research activities, including technology transfer, in universities and research institutes. The results of ANVUR's evaluation determines the allocation of public funding to universities. Interestingly, its own work is subject to evaluation, by a periodically convened committee of international experts appointed by the Ministry of Education, University and Research.

9.7.3 REPRISE

REPRISE was established at the Italian Ministry of Education, University and Research (MIUR). It is a register of Italian and foreign independent scientific experts. The register is made up of four sections: fundamental research; competitive industry and better society research; scientific culture spread; and administrative and accounting auditing and economic-financial assessment.

So, Italy is also moving from an assessment system that concentrated on bibliometrics of journal papers to a greater emphasis on the creation of society impact. One of its problems is the potential overlap between the various quality review systems.

9.8 Ireland

According to Murphy [17], Ireland recognises the potential for the science and innovation system to drive economic growth, and so it continues to increase its level of investment in scientific research. Universities and research funders face the challenge of selecting research projects and programmes that are aligned with national priorities and can have the most impact on the economy and society as a whole. The position of funding along the output-to-impact continuum and the methods of impact review vary across funders. Nonetheless, there is growing commonality in relation to the definition of impact and the importance of placing impact at the heart of funding strategies [17].

Science Foundation Ireland (SFI) is Ireland's largest scientific funding agency. In its strategy 'Agenda 2020' its vision is by 2020 to be the best science funding agency in the world at creating impact from excellent research and demonstrating clear value for money invested. While scientific excellence continues to be at the core of all funding decisions, in recent years impact has gained equal focus across all significant funding programmes. As with the REF, SFI recognises that impact may be short or long term, non-linear, difficult to measure and, perhaps more importantly, that there are many types of impact, not just economic or commercial.

SFI classifies the impacts of scientific research according to eight pillars [17]. These are Economic and Commercial; Societal; International Engagement; Impacts on Public Policy, Services and Regulations; Health and Well-Being; Environmental; Impact on Professional Services; Impacts on Human Capacity. Cross-cutting themes in these pillars are creating new products, processes, policies or behaviours; improving efficiency and efficacy of existing practices, policies, etc.; and building resilience, sustainability and reducing risk. It is against these pillars that the potential and actual impact are assessed [18].

Encouraged by the SFI's focus on research impact, many Irish universities have developed Impact Frameworks dealing with, Economic,

Societal, Environmental, Human Capacity and Health Impacts. While impact at a research project level is important, a partnership approach sees SFI working with universities to evaluate and communicate the longer term impacts of scientific research. The end result is a growing collection of impact case studies arising from the research base that point to a highly productive and impactful research sector [17].

9.9 Spain

Jimenez-Contreras et al. [19] discussed the evolution of research in Spain over the previous quarter of a century. They showed how from 1982 to 1991 the government began to invest heavily in research by implementing a set of legal measures and the creation of new research posts. However, it was only from 1989 that Spain began to take research assessment seriously. As in other countries, this was because Spanish research funding is highly dependent on the public sector. To get a feel for the return on research investment, the Government created the Comisión Nacional de Evaluación de la Actividad Investigadora (CNEAI). In English this is the National Commission for the Evaluation of Research Performance. This led to the maintenance of, and an increase in, the rate of research activity in Spain. As with the REF, the CNEAI has research performance reviews every 6 years. From 2019, it provided monetary incentives to researchers who submit 'evidence of impact and influence" of their research "on social and economic matters'.

9.10 Conclusion

Unfortunately, due to issues of space, it was not possible to provide a comprehensive discussion of all countries that are focusing on societal impact as a major component in their review of research quality. Nonetheless, from the above, it can be seen that many countries have kept a close eye on the UK REF process, especially with regard to the assessment of research impact. From these exam-

ples, and from work undertaken by the OECD [20], it is obvious that there is growing demand for the assessment of impact from publicly funded research. The assessment is increasing and changing from evaluating the quality of research via peer review, to assessing the outcome, output and impact of public research.

Lessons learned from this include the realisation that social/economic impacts require new metrics and approaches and stakeholder involvement as well as new communication channels to decision makers, to agents, and to stakeholders. Impact assessment must also balance the tension that exists between scientific relevance and social/economic impacts. This overview of research assessment in different countries demonstrates that the assessment of impact is an issue of growing interest, mainly in those countries (EU, Canada, Australia, USA) that invest more in research.

9.11 Summary

Impact assessment is becoming part and parcel of research evaluation across the globe. The rationale for this is becoming clearer as are policy needs for assessing the impacts of strategic research. However, assessing impacts is neither straightforward nor easy especially as regards demonstrating causality. Many of the societal, cultural or environmental impacts are difficult to measure or evaluate. Nevertheless, methodological difficulties should not stand in the way of efforts to undertake such evaluation. New and useful impact assessment approaches are being developed but international comparability remains a challenge [20]. Considering that research is increasingly being conducted by teams across countries, a solution to this is a priority. One solution, that received much publicity after the 2014 REF, was that the UK should sell its REF assessment exercise to other countries.

The examples provided in this chapter show some trends. One is the shifting focus from journal papers and citations to societal impact. Another is the use of impact case studies to provide a qualitative and quantitative description of impact. Yet another is the move away from the starting point of economic impact to impact on culture, health, quality of life, etc. Where most of these research assessment systems differ from the REF is that they are focused almost entirely on having positive impact in their own country. In contrast, the REF lauds the UK's ability to have impact nationally and internationally. This was evidenced in REF 2014, where UK research had impact in every country in the world. Another difference is the fact that, unlike the UK, most countries do not tie the performance in research assessment exercises with funding allocation. However, this is also to change.

References

1. Goodall J. Hope for animals and their world: how endangered species are being rescued from the brink. New York, NY: Grand Central Publishing; 2009. ISBN 0-446-58177-1.
2. Digital Science. The societal and economic impacts of academic research international perspectives on good practice and managing evidence; 2016. https://www.digital-science.com/resources/digital-research-reports/digital-research-report-societal-economic-impacts-academic-research/.
3. Duryea M, Hochman M, Parfitt A. Measuring the impact of research. Research Global. 2007; 27:8–9. http://www.atn.edu.au/docs/Research%20 Global%20-%20Measuring%20the%20impact%20 of%20research.pdf.
4. ARC. Engagement and impact. Canberra, ACT: Australian Research Council; 2020. https://www.arc. gov.au/engagement-and-impact-assessment.
5. KEF. Knowledge exchange framework. Research England; 2020. https://re.ukri.org/knowledge-exchange/ knowledge-exchange-framework/.
6. Muirhead, D. Willetts, J. Crawford, J. Hutchison, J. Smales, P. From Evidence to Impact: Development contribution of Australian Aid funded research: A study based on research undertaken through the Australian Development Research Awards Scheme 2007–2016. 2017. https://rdinetwork.org.au/wpcontent/uploads/2018/01/G2335_ADRAS-EXEC-SUMMARY_WEB_V2-1.pdf (accessed Sept 2020).
7. O'Sullivan M. Hong Kong's RAE is a colonial throwback. The Times Higher; 2018. https:// www.timeshighereducation.com/opinion/ hong-kongs-rae-colonial-throwback.
8. Canadian Academy of Health Sciences. Canadian Academy of Health Sciences Making an impact: a preferred framework and indicators to measure returns on investment in health research. Ottawa, ON:

Canadian Academy of Health Sciences; 2009. http:// www.cahs-acss.ca/e/pdfs/ROI_FullReport.pdf.
9. RIC Research Impact Canada; 2020. http:// researchimpact.ca/research-with-impact/.
10. Lane J, Bertuzzi S. Measuring the results of science investments. Science. 2011;331(6018):678–80. https://doi.org/10.1126/science.1201865. PMID 21310987.
11. The Bellagio Statement. Roadmap to measuring the results of investments in science: The Bellagio Statement; 2011. https://www.semanticscholar.org/ paper/EU%2FU.S.-Roadmap-to-measuring-the-results-of-in-the-Bertuzzi-Brandtner/d05be06c89bb7 196d7280377ea8d7ce23cb9914e?p2df
12. Sivertsen G. Unique, but still best practice? The Research Excellence Framework (REF) from an international perspective. Palgrave Commun. 2017;3:17078. https://doi.org/10.1057/ palcomms.2017.78.
13. Courea E. Redefine impact or face catastrophe – commission told. Research Fortnight; 2017. https:// www.researchprofessional.com/0/rr/news/europe/ horizon-2020/2017/10/Redefine-impact-or-face-catastrophe-Commission-told.html?utm_ medium=email&utm_source=rpMailing&utm_ campaign=personalNewsDailyUpdate_2017-10-13#sthash.XqIsCWm7.dpuf.
14. LERU. 23 leading universities pushing the frontiers of innovative research; 2020. https://www.leru.org/.
15. Barker KE, Cox D, Spaapen J, Van der Meulen B, Molas Gallert J, de Jong S, Tong P. Final report on social impacts of research. Manchester: The University of Manchester; 2011. https://www.research.manchester.ac.uk/portal/files/33083211/FULL_TEXT.PDF.
16. Reale E, Barbara A, Costantini A. Peer review for the evaluation of academic research: lessons from the Italian experience. Res Eval. 2007;16(3):216–28. https://doi.org/10.3152/095820207X227501.
17. Murphy L. Ireland – a proposed national system for assessing impact. In: Digital Science the societal and economic impacts of academic research international perspectives on good practice and managing evidence; 2016. https://www.digital-science.com/resources/dig-ital-research-reports/digital-research-report-societal-economic-impacts-academic-research/.
18. SFI. Research impact. Learn more about research impacts, preparing impact statements and reporting impacts. Dublin: Science Foundation Ireland; 2020. https://www.sfi.ie/funding/award-management/ research-impact/.
19. Jimenez-Contreras E, de Moya Anegon F, Delgado Lopez-Cozar E. The evolution of research activity in Spain: the impact of the National Commission for the Evaluation of Research Activity (CNEAI). Res Policy. 2003;32(1):123–42.
20. OECD. Enhancing research performance through evaluation, impact assessment and priority setting; 2009. https://www.oecd.org/sti/inno/Enhancing-Public-Research-Performance.pdf.

Appendix

Appendix A: Engagement with External Stakeholders for Research Impact

Who are the actual and potential research users?	Who, among your colleagues, are already working with them?	Where are the actual and potential research users?
i…	i…	i…
ii…	ii…	ii…
iii…	iii…	iii…
When in the best time to engage with them?	What are their interests, priorities and needs?	What is in it for them; how will they benefit?
i…	i…	i…
ii…	ii…	ii…
iii…	iii…	iii…
What are your objectives from this engagement?	What methods will you use to access and engage with them?	What resources will you need to create meaningful engagement?
i…	i…	i…
ii…	ii…	ii…
iii…	iii…	iii…
How do you align your objectives with their priorities?	What are the main barriers to successful engagement?	How do you ensure long-term engagement?
i…	i…	i…
ii…	ii…	ii…
iii…	iii…	iii…

© The Editor(s) (if applicable) and The Author(s),
under exclusive license to Springer Nature Switzerland AG 2021
H. P. McKenna, *Research Impact*, https://doi.org/10.1007/978-3-030-57028-6

Appendix B: Research Impact Case Study Checklist

Criterion	Y/N
• Adherence to the word limit and number of pages	
• The staff names and roles are specified	
• The period when the staff were employed in the submitting university is clear	
• Clarify if this is a continued impact case study	
• Clear indication that underpinning research was at least two star quality	
• Include up to six references to the underpinning research	
• Include research funding amounts and sources	
• Each impact's reach is clear	
• Each impact's significance is clear	
• The impact(s) are strongly connected to the underpinning research	
• The impact(s) are strongly connected to the submitting UoAs	
• The underpinning research adhered to the output assessment timeframe	
• The impact occurred in the designated impact timeframe	
• The corroborating sources can confirm the impact claims	
• Quantitative data are provided to support the qualitative narrative	

Appendix C: Creating Impact Through Public Engagement

Who are the people or companies that you need to connect with to create impact?	Has your university already got links with them?	Where and when will the event take place?
i…	i…	i…
ii…	ii…	ii…
iii…	iii…	iii…
When is the best time to present to them and how will you present?	Why should they be interested in your research findings?	What are the main messages you want to get across?
i…	i…	i…
ii…	ii…	ii…
iii…	iii…	iii…
How do you inform them that you are seeking to change their views or behaviours?	If required, how do you ensure you followed GDPR legislation?	What support and resources will you need to engage and follow up?
i…	i…	i…
ii…	ii…	ii…
iii…	iii…	iii…
Once the event is finished, how do you follow up?	What data do you need to collect to demonstrate impact?	What methods will you use to collect the evidence of impact?
i…	i…	i…
ii…	ii…	ii…
iii…	iii…	iii…

Appendix D: Research Impact Through Changing Policy

Who are the policymakers you need to influence?	What is the best way to access them?	How can you show them that that this will be to their benefit?
i…	i…	i…
ii…	ii…	ii…
iii…	iii…	iii…
When in the best time/place to engage with them?	Can your research fit with their interests, priorities and hobbies?	How can you get your message across in a succinct way?
i…	i…	i…
ii…	ii…	ii…
iii…	iii…	iii…
Will social media have a part to play?	What policy do you want to create, influence or change?	What will you need to see in a policy to provide you with evidence of success?
i…	i…	i…
ii…	ii…	ii…
iii…	iii…	iii…
What testimonial details do you need from ministers or officials?	What are the main barriers to your success?	If the minister/official moved on, what is your alternative plan?
i…	i…	i…
ii…	ii…	ii…
iii…	iii…	iii…